Facial Paralysis

Editors

JON-PAUL PEPPER

TRAVIS T. TOLLEFSON

FACIAL PLASTIC SURGERY CLINICS OF NORTH AMERICA

www.facialplastic.theclinics.com

Consulting Editor
J. REGAN THOMAS

August 2021 • Volume 29 • Number 3

ELSEVIER

1600 John F. Kennedy Boulevard • Suite 1800 • Philadelphia, Pennsylvania, 19103-2899

http://www.theclinics.com

FACIAL PLASTIC SURGERY CLINICS OF NORTH AMERICA Volume 29, Number 3
August 2021 ISSN 1064-7406, ISBN-13: 978-0-323-75632-7

Editor: Stacy Eastman
Developmental Editor: Ann Gielou M. Posedio

Facial Plastic Surgery Clinics of North America (ISSN 1064-7406) is published quarterly by Elsevier Inc., 360 Park Avenue South, New York, NY 10010-1710. Months of issue are February, May, August, and November. Business and Editorial Offices: 1600 John F. Kennedy Blvd., Suite 1800, Philadelphia, PA 19103-2899. Periodicals postage paid at New York, NY, and additional mailing offices. Subscription prices are $412.00 per year (US individuals), $895.00 per year (US institutions), $459.00 per year (Canadian individuals), $944.00 per year (Canadian institutions), $546.00 per year (foreign individuals), $944.00 per year (foreign institutions), $100.00 per year (US students), $100.00 per year (Canadian students), and $255.00 per year (foreign students). Foreign air speed delivery is included in all *Clinics* subscription prices. All prices are subject to change without notice. POSTMASTER: Send address changes to *Facial Plastic Surgery Clinics*, Elsevier Health Sciences Division, Subscription Customer Service, 3251 Riverport Lane, Maryland Heights, MO 63043. **Customer service: 1-800-654-2452 (US and Canada); 1-314-447-8871 (outside US and Canada); Fax: 314-447-8029; E-mail: journalscustomerservice-usa@elsevier.com (for print support); journalsonlinesupport-usa@elsevier.com (for online support).**

Reprints. For copies of 100 or more of articles in this publication, please contact the Commercial Reprints Department, Elsevier Inc., 360 Park Avenue South, New York, NY 10010-1710. Tel.: 212-633-3874; Fax: 212-633-3820; E-mail: reprints@elsevier.com.

Facial Plastic Surgery Clinics of North America is covered in *MEDLINE/PubMed* (*Index Medicus*).

Contributors

CONSULTING EDITOR

J. REGAN THOMAS, MD
Professor, Facial Plastic and Reconstructive
Surgery, Department of Otolaryngology–Head
and Neck Surgery, Northwestern University
Feinberg School of Medicine, Chicago, Illinois,
USA

EDITORS

JON-PAUL PEPPER, MD
Director, Stanford Facial Nerve Center,
Assistant Professor, Division of Facial Plastic
and Reconstructive Surgery, Department of
Otolaryngology–Head and Neck Surgery,
Stanford University School of Medicine,
Stanford, California, USA

TRAVIS T. TOLLEFSON, MD, MPH
Professor and Director, Facial Plastic and
Reconstructive Surgery, Department of
Otolaryngology–Head and Neck Surgery,
University of California, Davis, Sacramento,
California, USA

AUTHORS

BABAK AZIZZADEH, MD, FACS
The Facial Paralysis Institute, Beverly Hills,
California, USA

GREGORY H. BORSCHEL, MD, FACS, FAAP
Division of Plastic and Reconstructive Surgery,
Hospital for Sick Children (SickKids), University
of Toronto, Toronto, Ontario, Canada

PATRICK J. BYRNE, MD, MBA
Chair, Head and Neck Institute, Cleveland
Clinic Foundation, Cleveland, Ohio

SIMEON C. DAESCHLER, MD
Neuroscience and Mental Health Program,
Hospital for Sick Children (SickKids), Toronto,
Ontario, Canada

ABEL P. DAVID, MD
Department of Otolaryngology–Head and Neck
Surgery, University of California, San
Francisco, San Francisco, California, USA

RAJ D. DEDHIA, MD
Department of Otolaryngology–Head and Neck
Surgery, The University of Tennessee Health
Science Center, Memphis, Tennessee, USA

ANDRES F. DOVAL, MD
Research Fellow, Institute for Reconstructive
Surgery, Houston Methodist Hospital,
Houston, Texas, USA

TESSA A. HADLOCK, MD
Division of Facial Plastic and Reconstructive
Surgery, Department of Otolaryngology,
Massachusetts Eye and Ear, Harvard Medical
School, Boston, Massachusetts, USA

NIKOLAUS HJELM, MD
The Facial Paralysis Institute, Beverly Hills,
California, USA

NATE JOWETT, MD
Department of Otolaryngology–Head and Neck
Surgery, Massachusetts Eye and Ear, Harvard
Medical School, Boston, Massachusetts, USA

JENNIFER C. KIM, MD
Associate Professor of Otolaryngology–Head and Neck Surgery, University Michigan Health Systems, Ann Arbor, Michigan, USA

MICHAEL J. KLEBUC, MD
Director of the Center for Facial Paralysis and Functional Restoration, Associate Clinical Professor of Plastic and Reconstructive Surgery, Institute for Reconstructive Surgery, Houston Methodist Hospital, Houston, Texas, USA; Weill Cornell School of Medicine, New York, New York, USA

PHILIP DANIEL KNOTT, MD
Professor and Director, Division of Facial Plastic and Reconstructive Surgery, Department of Otolaryngology–Head and Neck Surgery, University of California, San Francisco, San Francisco, California, USA

G. NINA LU, MD
Assistant Professor, Department of Otolaryngology, Division of Facial Plastic and Reconstructive Surgery, University of Washington, Seattle, Washington, USA

SOFIA LYFORD-PIKE, MD
Department of Otolaryngology–Head and Neck Surgery, University of Minnesota, Minneapolis, Minnesota, USA

DAMIR MATIC, MD
Associate Professor, Division of Plastic and Reconstructive Surgery, Department of Surgery, Schulich School of Medicine and Dentistry, University of Western Ontario, Victoria Hospital, London, Ontario, Canada

MATTHEW Q. MILLER, MD
Division of Facial Plastic and Reconstructive Surgery, Department of Otolaryngology, Massachusetts Eye and Ear, Harvard Medical School, Boston, Massachusetts, USA

JASON C. NELLIS, MD
Department of Otolaryngology–Head and Neck Surgery, University of Minnesota, Minneapolis, Minnesota, USA; Edina, Minnesota, USA

TYLER S. OKLAND, MD
Department of Otolaryngology–Head and Neck Surgery, Stanford University School of Medicine, Stanford, California, USA

SAMUEL L. OYER, MD
Associate Professor, Facial Plastic and Reconstructive Surgery, Department of Otolaryngology–Head and Neck Surgery, University of Virginia, Charlottesville, Virginia, USA

KRISHNA G. PATEL, MD, PhD
Professor, Facial Plastic and Reconstructive Surgery, Department of Otolaryngology–Head and Neck Surgery, Medical University of South Carolina, Charleston, South Carolina, USA

JON-PAUL PEPPER, MD
Director, Stanford Facial Nerve Center, Assistant Professor, Division of Facial Plastic and Reconstructive Surgery, Department of Otolaryngology–Head and Neck Surgery, Stanford University School of Medicine, Stanford, California, USA

ROBERTO PINEDA II, MD
Department of Ophthalmology, Massachusetts Eye and Ear, Harvard Medical School, Boston, Massachusetts, USA

JASON D. POU, MD
Physician, Facial Plastic and Reconstructive Surgery, Department of Otolaryngology–Head and Neck Surgery, Ochsner Medical Center, New Orleans, Louisiana, USA

ALMOAIDBELLAH RAMMAL, MD
Clinical Fellow, Department of Otolaryngology–Head and Neck Surgery, Western University, Victoria Hospital, London Health Science Centre, London, Ontario, Canada; Department of Otolaryngology–Head and Neck Surgery, King Abdul-Aziz University, Jeddah, Saudi Arabia

RAHUL SETH, MD
Associate Professor and Co-Fellowship Director, Division of Facial Plastic and Reconstructive Surgery, Department of Otolaryngology–Head and Neck Surgery, University of California, San Francisco, San Francisco, California, USA

TAHA Z. SHIPCHANDLER, MD
Department of Otolaryngology–Head and Neck Surgery, Indiana University School of Medicine, Indiana, USA

TRAVIS T. TOLLEFSON, MD, MPH
Professor and Director, Facial Plastic and
Reconstructive Surgery, Department of
Otolaryngology–Head and Neck Surgery,
University of California, Davis, Sacramento,
California, USA

AMY S. XUE, MD
Institute for Reconstructive Surgery, Houston
Methodist Hospital, Houston, Texas, USA

SHIAYIN F. YANG, MD
Assistant Professor of Otolaryngology–Head
and Neck Surgery, Vanderbilt University
Medical Center, Nashville, Tennessee, USA

JOHN YOO, MD
Professor, Department of Otolaryngology–
Head and Neck Surgery, Western University,
Victoria Hospital, London Health Science
Centre, London, Ontario, Canada

**RONALD ZUKER, MD, FRCSC, FACS, FAAP,
FRCSEd(Hon)**
Division of Plastic and Reconstructive Surgery,
Hospital for Sick Children (SickKids), University
of Toronto, Toronto, Ontario, Canada

Contributors

TRAVIS T. TOLLEFSON, MD, MPH
Professor and Director, Facial Plastic and
Reconstructive Surgery, Department of
Otolaryngology-Head and Neck Surgery,
University of California, Davis, Sacramento,
California, USA

AMY S. XUE, MD
Institute for Reconstructive Surgery, Houston
Methodist Hospital, Houston, Texas, USA

SHIAYIN F. YANG, MD
Assistant Professor, a Otolaryngology-Head
and Neck Surgery, Vanderbilt University
Medical Center, Nashville, Tennessee, USA

JOHN YOO, MD
Professor, Department of Otolaryngology-
Head and Neck Surgery, Western University,
Victoria Hospital, London Health Sciences
Centre, London, Ontario, Canada

RONALD ZUKER, MD, FRCSC, FACS, FAAP,
FRCSEd(Hon)
Division of Plastic and Reconstructive Surgery,
Hospital for Sick Children (SickKids), University
of Toronto, Toronto, Ontario, Canada

Contents

Foreword: Steps Forward: Contemporary Treatment of Facial Paralysis　　　xiii

J. Regan Thomas

Preface: Steps Forward: Contemporary Treatment of Facial Paralysis　　　xv

Jon-Paul Pepper and Travis T. Tollefson

Perceptions of Patients with Facial Paralysis: Predicting Social Implications and Setting Goals　　　369

Sofia Lyford-Pike and Jason C. Nellis

The goal of this article is to better understand the social impact of facial paralysis. Patients with facial paralysis may suffer from impaired social interactions, disruption of self-concept, psychological distress, and decreased overall quality of life. Vigilance in detecting patients suffering from mental health issues may result in providing early referral for psychological evaluation and psychosocial support resources complementing facial reanimation treatment.

Static Sling Options for Facial Paralysis: Now Versus 10 Years Ago　　　375

Almoaidbellah Rammal, John Yoo, and Damir Matic

Static facial sling procedures are one of many facial reanimation options to address long-standing and irreversible facial paralysis. The primary goals of static reanimation are to provide symmetry at rest and improve static function at repose. Choosing the best option depends on patient factors, such as age, comorbidities, and injury factors. Different materials are available for static sling surgery; we believe autologous tendon offers the most reliable and long-lasting results. Static suspension procedures provide immediate results, improved resting position, and can augment other techniques. This article discusses available options for static reanimations to address the eye complex, midface, and mouth.

Temporalis Tendon Transfer Versus Gracilis Free Muscle Transfer: When and Why?　　　383

G. Nina Lu and Patrick J. Byrne

Temporalis tendon transfer (T3) and gracilis free muscle transfer (GFMT) are popular techniques in lower facial rehabilitation when reinnervation techniques are unavailable. T3 involves a single-stage outpatient procedure resulting in immediate improvement in resting symmetry and a volitional smile. GFMT allows a spontaneous smile, customized vectors, and increased excursion but requires longer surgical time, a delay before movement, and specialized equipment. Ultimately, shared decision making between the clinician and patient should focus on the patient's goals and unique medical condition.

Reinnervation with Selective Nerve Grafting from Multiple Donor Nerves　　　389

Shiayin F. Yang and Jennifer C. Kim

 Video content accompanies this article at http://www.facialplastic.theclinics.com.

Nerve substitution is an important tool in facial reanimation. The goal is to reinnervate the distal facial nerve and musculature using an alternative cranial nerve in order to achieve facial movement, symmetry, and tone. Multiple donor nerves have been used for nerve transfer procedures, the most common being hypoglossal, masseteric, and cross-facial nerve graft. Each donor nerve has its advantages and disadvantages. Multiinnervation uses the use of multiple donor nerves in order to leverage the benefits while balancing the pitfalls of each nerve. The nerve transfer depends on the type of nerve injury, time since injury, and patient factors.

Dual Nerve Transfer for Facial Reanimation   397

Tyler S. Okland and Jon-Paul Pepper

 Video content accompanies this article at http://www.facialplastic.theclinics.com.

This article describes a method of performing a dual nerve transfer procedure and provides illustrative cases for analysis and discussion. Clinical indications, technical pearls, and pitfalls are discussed. Dual nerve transfer for facial reanimation efficiently combines the strengths of the hypoglossal and masseteric nerve transfers and builds on existing nerve transfer techniques.

Facial Reanimation and Reconstruction of the Radical Parotidectomy   405

Abel P. David, Rahul Seth, and Philip Daniel Knott

Radical parotidectomy may result from treating advanced parotid malignancies invading the facial nerve. Survival is often enhanced with multimodality treatment protocols, including postoperative radiation therapy. In addition to the reconstructive challenge of restoring facial nerve function, patients may be left with a significant cervicofacial concavity and inadequate skin coverage. This should be addressed with stable vascularized tissue that is resistant to radiation-induced atrophy. This article describes a comprehensive strategy, includes the use of the anterolateral thigh free flap, the temporalis regional muscle transfer, motor nerve to vastus lateralis grafts, nerve to masseter transfer, and fascia lata grafts for static suspension.

Lessons from Gracilis Free Tissue Transfer for Facial Paralysis: Now versus 10 Years Ago   415

Matthew Q. Miller and Tessa A. Hadlock

Outcomes following free gracilis muscle transfer have steadily improved during the past decade. Areas for continued improvement include re-creating natural smile vectors, improving midface symmetry, minimizing scarring, improving spontaneity, and increasing reliability using various neural sources. Outcome standardization, pooled data collection, and remote data acquisition methods will facilitate comparative effectiveness research and continued surgical advancements.

Strategies to Improve Cross-Face Nerve Grafting in Facial Paralysis   423

Simeon C. Daeschler, Ronald Zuker, and Gregory H. Borschel

Cross-face nerve grafting enables the reanimation of the contralateral hemiface in unilateral facial palsy and may recover a spontaneous smile. This chapter discusses various clinically applicable strategies to increase the chances for good functional outcomes by maintaining the viability of the neural pathway and target muscle, increasing the number of reinnervating nerve fibers and selecting functionally compatible donor nerve branches. Adopting those strategies may help to further improve patient outcomes in facial reanimation surgery.

Dual Innervation of Free Functional Muscle Flaps in Facial Paralysis   431

Michael J. Klebuc, Amy S. Xue, and Andres F. Doval

Dual innervation in free muscle flap facial reanimation has been used to create a functional synergy between the powerful commissure excursion that can be achieved with the masseter nerve and the spontaneity that can be derived from a cross-face nerve graft. The gracilis has been the most frequently used muscle flap, and multiple combinations of neurorrhaphies have been described, including the masseter to the obturator (end-to-end) combined with a cross-face nerve graft to the obturator (end-to-side) and vice versa. Single and staged approaches have been reported. Minimally, dual innervation is as effective as using the motor nerve to masseter alone.

Treating Nasal Valve Collapse in Facial Paralysis: What I Do Differently   439

Jason D. Pou, Krishna G. Patel, and Samuel L. Oyer

Patients with facial paralysis require a systematic zonal assessment. One frequently overlooked region is the effect of facial paralysis on nasal airflow. Patients with flaccid paralysis experience increased weight of the cheek and loss of muscle tone in the ala and sidewall; this significantly contributes to nasal valve narrowing and collapse. These specific findings are often not adequately corrected with traditional functional rhinoplasty-grafting techniques. Flaccid paralysis typically results in inferomedial displacement of the alar base, which must be restored with suspension techniques to fully treat the nasal obstruction. Multiple surgical options exist and are discussed in this article.

Eyelid Coupling Using a Modified Tarsoconjunctival Flap in Facial Paralysis   447

Raj D. Dedhia, Taha Z. Shipchandler, and Travis T. Tollefson

Eyelid coupling using the modified tarsoconjunctival flap is an effective treatment for paralytic ectropion. Eyelid position and quality of life can be improved in patients with flaccid facial paralysis using these eyelid coupling procedures. The modified tarsoconjunctival flap can obscure the lateral visual field by coupling the eyelids, but without distortion of the canthal angle and eyelid margin. The procedure is often coupled with a lateral canthoplasty or canthopexy to address horizontal laxity of the lower eyelid. Collecting standardized outcome measures will help establish the ideal treatment paradigm of paralytic eyelid malposition.

Modified Selective Neurectomy: A New Paradigm in the Management of Facial Palsy with Synkinesis   453

Babak Azizzadeh and Nikolaus Hjelm

All patients with postparalytic facial paralysis are at risk of developing synkinesis due to aberrant nerve regeneration. Synkinesis can result in smile dysfunction, tension, and eyelid aperture narrowing due to overactive and uncoordinated muscle activity. When the synkinesis causes an asymmetric smile, there are several treatment modalities including neurotoxin, neuromuscular retraining, and surgery. Modified selective neurectomy of the facial nerve is a treatment option that potentially can improve the smile mechanism by reducing the activity of counterproductive facial muscles while preserving the natural neural pathway.

Corneal and Facial Sensory Neurotization in Trigeminal Anesthesia   **459**

Nate Jowett and Roberto Pineda II

Trigeminal anesthesia may yield blindness and facial disfigurement, secondary to neurotrophic keratopathy and trigeminal trophic syndrome. This article summarizes contemporary medical and emerging surgical approaches for the therapeutic management of this rare and devastating disease state.

FACIAL PLASTIC SURGERY CLINICS OF NORTH AMERICA

FORTHCOMING ISSUES

November 2021
Facial Plastic Surgery Procedures in the Non-Caucasian Population
Yong Ju Jang, *Editor*

February 2022
Modern Approaches to Facial and Athletic Injuries
J. David Kriet and Clinton D. Humphrey, *Editors*

May 2022
Facial and Nasal Anatomy
Sebastian Cotofana, *Editor*

RECENT ISSUES

May 2021
Oculoplastic Surgery
John B. Holds and Guy G. Massry, *Editors*

February 2021
Preservation Rhinoplasty
Sam P. Most, *Editor*

November 2020
Day-to-Day Challenges in Facial Plastic Surgery
William H. Truswell, *Editor*

SERIES OF RELATED INTEREST

Clinics in Plastic Surgery
https://www.plasticsurgery.theclinics.com
Otolaryngologic Clinics
https://www.oto.theclinics.com
Dermatologic Clinics
https://www.derm.theclinics.com

THE CLINICS ARE AVAILABLE ONLINE!
Access your subscription at:
www.theclinics.com

Foreword
Steps Forward: Contemporary Treatment of Facial Paralysis

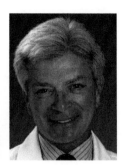

J. Regan Thomas, MD
Consulting Editor

Facial paralysis has a dramatic effect on the patient's self-image and well-being, their social interaction, and multiple aspects of facial function, creating a variety of clinical issues. Treatment and correction of facial paralysis is an extremely important, although often complicated, component of facial plastic surgery.

There are multiple procedures and techniques to treat facial paralysis depending on the patient's presentation of the condition and the surgeon's experience and preference. There are a variety of surgical options for the treatment of facial paralysis, and there has been notable progress in improving outcomes and results in recent years.

This issue presents a variety of techniques and surgical approaches to treating this challenging condition. Dr Pepper and Dr Tollefson, both experienced practitioners in treatment of facial paralysis, have assembled a group of expert authors to describe and discuss their techniques and experienced results in facial paralysis treatment. A variety of approaches are described in detail, and the reader will benefit from insights into numerous

methods of dealing with this challenging clinical situation.

Treatment of facial paralysis continues to evolve and change to the benefit of the treating surgeons and the improvement of outcomes for this group of patients. This issue of *Facial Plastic Surgery Clinics of North America*, which has been organized by Drs Pepper and Tollefson, will provide a useful resource and reference for our specialty readership. This assembled group of authors and the descriptions and explanations of their approaches and techniques will contribute to the knowledge base of our specialty at large.

J. Regan Thomas, MD
Facial Plastic and Reconstructive Surgery
Department of Otolaryngology–
Head and Neck Surgery
Northwestern University
School of Medicine
60 East Delaware Place
Chicago, IL 60611, USA

E-mail address:
jreganthomas@gmail.com

Facial Plast Surg Clin N Am 29 (2021) xiii
https://doi.org/10.1016/j.fsc.2021.04.002
1064-7406/21/

Preface
Steps Forward: Contemporary Treatment of Facial Paralysis

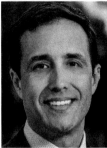

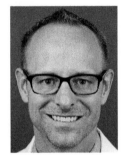

Jon-Paul Pepper, MD   Travis T. Tollefson, MD, MPH
Editors

The treatment of facial paralysis is demanding and multifaceted and is a collaborative surgical effort that requires both surgical innovation and rigorous assessment of outcomes. Although there are certainly patterns in patient presentation, patients with facial paralysis often have unique mixtures of clinical problems. As such, no single procedure can claim reliable and comprehensive restoration of normal movement in all cases. It is perhaps for this reason that surgical treatment of facial paralysis is such a dynamic area, with continuous surgical refinement and new techniques. Importantly, this spirit of active improvement has resulted in more than just new techniques. There has been notable progress in the treatment of facial paralysis, with improved and more reliable outcomes, and overall a greater number of *effective* surgical options. This breadth requires that surgeons who treat this disorder stay current on the many treatment options available. To address this need, this issue represents a state-of-the-art collection of surgical techniques and treatment considerations that are proven to be effective or are particularly innovative and trending toward more widespread adoption.

It is impossible to include all the authors who have helped move this field forward. Therefore, this issue should be viewed as a sampling of contemporary techniques that can serve as a foundation for further exploration. The science of facial paralysis treatment has been greatly impacted by the widespread adoption of patient-reported outcome measures and objective assessments of facial symmetry and movement. Several of the senior authors in this issue, in particular, Dr Tessa Hadlock, have been instrumental in leading and encouraging our community in this regard.

If this collection of work is examined closely over its entirety, one will see subtle signs of disagreement between expert practitioners. This is a testament to the ever-adapting nature of this field and the reality that no technique is yet comprehensive. While there is no "silver bullet" treatment, there is certainly an impressive array of effective tools.

We owe sincere thanks to this highly acclaimed group of surgeons. We also owe special thanks to our patients, who continue to place their trust in our hands. For them, we continue the challenging but wonderful work of facial paralysis treatment

Facial Plast Surg Clin N Am 29 (2021) xv–xvi
https://doi.org/10.1016/j.fsc.2021.04.001
1064-7406/21/© 2021 Published by Elsevier Inc.

with high enthusiasm and a clear sense of purpose.

Jon-Paul Pepper, MD
Stanford Facial Nerve Center
Division of Facial Plastic and
Reconstructive Surgery
Department of Otolaryngology–
Head and Neck Surgery
Stanford University School of Medicine
801 Welch Road
Stanford, CA 94305, USA

Travis T. Tollefson, MD, MPH
Facial Plastic and Reconstructive Surgery
Department of Otolaryngology–
Head and Neck Surgery
University of California Davis
2521 Stockton Boulevard, Suite 7200
Sacramento, CA 95817, USA

E-mail addresses:
jpepper@stanford.edu (J.-P. Pepper)
tttollefson@ucdavis.edu (T.T. Tollefson)

Perceptions of Patients with Facial Paralysis
Predicting Social Implications and Setting Goals

Sofia Lyford-Pike, MD[a],*, Jason C. Nellis, MD[b,c]

KEYWORDS

- Facial paralysis • Social impact • Psychosocial heath • Quality of life • Self-concept
- Social perceptions • Psychological distress

KEY POINTS

- Patients with facial paralysis suffer significant morbidity in social functioning because of the observed deformity at rest and ineffective movement. They are perceived as less attractive, having a more negative affect, and having a lower quality of life by observers in society.
- Individuals with facial paralysis may suffer from reduced self-esteem, increased anxiety, worse depression, and reduced quality of life.
- In treating patients with facial paralysis, social well-being should be an important consideration by the provider. The degree of facial dysfunction is predictive of the degree of casual observer perceived disfigurement, and thus, the social burden of the condition.
- Facial reanimation may assist in decreasing the psychosocial morbidity of facial paralysis.
- Early detection of mental health issues in patients with facial paralysis may improve overall care of this patient population.

BACKGROUND
Role of the Face

As an important factor in social interactions, the human face provides nonverbal cues regarding one's identity, sex, age, race, affect, and overall health.[1] Inferences are made by observers within 100 to 200 milliseconds of exposure to the face. These inferences are made from both static features of the face, such as attractiveness (composed of age, symmetry, sexually dimorphic shape cues, averageness, and skin color/texture) and disfigurement. This inference is evolutionarily rooted in humans in order to judge reproductive fitness of others and to identify threats. Facial movement is also fundamental in the interpersonal exchange between individuals. Individuals engaging in social interaction subconsciously mirror each other's facial expressions, resulting in emotional contagion and tacit psychosocial perceptions.[2] In addition, participants in the social exchange use facial expression to foster coherence and integration of information and emotions, such as interest or apprehension.[1,2]

Patients who develop facial deformity sustain a loss of physical function, such as the inability to speak or eat, and notably psychosocial function related to negative social perceptions. An example of such facial deformity is facial paralysis, which impairs facial movement, resulting in resting asymmetry that becomes highlighted when engaging in social interactions.

a Department of Otolaryngology–Head and Neck Surgery, University of Minnesota, 500 Harvard Street, Minneapolis, MN 55455, USA; b Department of Otolaryngology–Head and Neck Surgery, University of Minnesota, Minneapolis, MN, USA; c 7373 France Avenue South #410, Edina, MN 55435, USA
* Corresponding author. 7373 France Avenue South #410, Edina, MN 55435.
E-mail address: lyfor009@umn.edu

Facial Plast Surg Clin N Am 29 (2021) 369–374
https://doi.org/10.1016/j.fsc.2021.03.008

A negative social bias against those with visual facial differences permeates various cultures and time. Shaw[3] described examples of global prejudice to individuals with facial deformity, such as mothers rejecting children with cleft lip, the King of Denmark in 1708 forbidding interaction with people with facial deformity, and African tribes prohibiting people with facial deformity from becoming chief.[4] Accordingly, patients with facial paralysis have impaired facial expression, resulting in negative social ramifications. This article aims to discuss the social implications of facial paralysis and provides a basis for improving patient care beyond treating physical function.

SOCIAL IMPLICATIONS OF FACIAL PARALYSIS

Psychology literature in the analysis of facial movements and expressions is vast. Studies have more specifically looked at how casual observers assess the faces of individuals with facial paralysis. Using infrared eye-gaze tracker technology to record observers gazing on paralyzed and normal faces, Ishii and colleagues[5] found that casual observers gaze on a paralyzed face differently, with greater attention to the mouth, compared with a normal face, especially when smiling. Furthermore, Helwig and colleagues[6] characterized using an anatomically realistic 3-dimensional facial tool to study the spatiotemporal properties of smiles. It was found that the amount of dental show should be balanced to the smile extent and mouth angle and that timing asymmetries of smile onset can be detrimental to smiling effectiveness.

Casual observers perceive static images of a paralyzed face as having a more negative affect display when compared with images of nonaffected faces.[7] When assessing videos of movement, observers perceived individuals with severe facial paralysis as much less happy than those with mild facial paralysis, demonstrating that observers misperceive a face lacking expression.[8] Beyond negatively impacting affect display, several studies found negative social perceptions across other domains. Ishii and colleagues[9] tasked casual observers to identify a paralyzed face and rate the attractiveness as compared with normal faces, finding that paralyzed faces were rated as significantly less attractive. In addition, a smiling expression from patients was found to be unnatural by observers.[10] Additional studies have found that patients with facial paralysis appear distressed, less trustworthy, less intelligent, and abnormal.[11] Interestingly, Li and colleagues[11] distinguished between the various isolated regional facial paralysis presentations, finding that isolated zygomatic nerve palsy (ie, inability to close eye) results in the highest social detriment, and frontal palsy has the lowest social detriment.

Observer perception is not congruent with individual self-perception. Observers rated the quality of life of patients with facial paralysis to be worse than the individual's own self-assessment.[12] In addition, studies have found that physician experts also perceive patients with facial paralysis as having reduced attractiveness, increased severity, and worse perceived quality of life compared with how patients perceive themselves.[13] In the context of an individual's self-concept, the social perception morbidity of facial paralysis has related negative impact on his or her psychological well-being.

Impact of Facial Paralysis on Patients

Acquired facial paralysis has a negative effect on an individual's psychological well-being. Several studies have investigated quality of life, depression, anxiety, and other psychosocial factors associated with facial paralysis. Ryzenman and colleagues[14] found that 30% of patients were significantly distressed by facial paralysis after acoustic neuroma surgery. In an effort to understand the effect of facial paralysis resulting from other causes, investigations have found that patients with facial paralysis after parotidectomy suffer a decrease of quality of life in the first 3 months, but quality of life does improve after 1 year. Nevertheless, most patients in the study had full recovery of nerve function by that time.[15,16] Also, patients with Bell palsy have been found to report lower quality of life compared with patients with facial paralysis after acoustic neuroma resection.[17] In examining other factors, studies have found that increased facial paralysis severity, younger age, and female gender are associated with worse psychosocial patient-reported scores.[18–20] Interestingly, these findings were not found in pediatric patients with congenital facial paralysis.[21]

Although various factors influence quality of life, psychological distress can be associated with facial paralysis and potentially related to the social implications. Fu and colleagues[22] and Bradbury and colleagues[23] surveyed patients with facial paralysis and found that 31% to 60% of patients had significant depression and anxiety.[24] Notably, patients with depression were more likely to be dissatisfied with reconstructive procedures. However, these studies had not compared the prevalence of depression compared with controls. A prospective observational study found patients with facial paralysis suffered from worse depression, especially if the severity was House-

Brackmann grade 3 or higher, lower mood, lower self-reported attractiveness, and lower quality of life compared with control patients.[20]

There are several evolutionarily engrained functions of facial expressions and affect. As related to psychosocial distress, it is suggested that the ability to express an emotion is related to an individual's ability to recognize emotion implying an additional hurdle for social interactions for these patients. For example, individuals who received botulinum toxin treatment of the "scowling" muscles, the procerus and corrugators, showed less activity in the amygdala (the emotional area of the brain) when viewing angry faces.[25] Similarly, patients with Moebius syndrome have been found to have difficulty recognizing facial identities and facial expressions.[26] In a similar way, the ability to express a facial emotion also intensifies the experience of that emotion. This "facial feedback," as described by Lewis[27] and Ekman,[28] results from a centrally generated facial expression, for example, smiling resulting in a positive mood and scowling resulting in a negative mood. Facial mimicry, the manner by which an individual reflects another's expression on their own face, is important for social interactions and is also attenuated.[29] Patients thus do not effectively communicate nonverbally with facial cues and also suffer challenges in interpreting those cues from and connecting with others.

SETTING PATIENT CARE GOALS

It is important that providers consider the social morbidity experienced by patients with facial paralysis and visual facial differences. The social dimension is one not often explored in the clinic setting, but is fundamental to the well-being of the individuals we treat. Treating these patients must go beyond corneal health, speech, and eating and must include treatments to minimize disfigurement and optimize nonverbal communication.

The first step is to discuss the social dimension in the consultation. We can now predict the social burden of the paralysis by the clinical degree of facial function[30]; this helps discuss and determine treatment goals with each individual patient.

When treating patients with facial paralysis, facial reanimation can achieve many goals. These goals include resting symmetry, eyelid closure for corneal protection, restoration of smile, improved brow posture, oral competence, and return of voluntary facial movement. For movement, the goal is to achieve spontaneous facial movement that is absent of synkinesis or mass movement. Beyond physical functions, understanding the potential psychosocial benefits, and limitations, of

facial reanimation facilitates discussions with patients about surgical interventions and rehabilitation to achieve the goals mentioned above.

Facial reanimation has been found to improve function in the psychosocial dimension. Several studies have aimed to understand how facial reanimation surgery restores normal facial function and improves social perceptions of patients with facial paralysis. Using eye-gaze tracking technology, a study found that facial reanimation surgery restores how observers gaze patterns to normal.[31] In a study comparing observer perceptions of patients having undergone surgery to treat facial paralysis, patients sustain a significant improvement in affect display, especially when smiling.[32] Furthermore, facial reanimation improves patient attractiveness, but does not return them completely to premorbid baseline as compared with controls.[33] A subsequent study found that observers highly value facial reanimation surgery with a mean willingness to pay per quality-adjusted life year of $10,167 for low-grade facial paralysis and $17,008 for high-grade facial paralysis.[34]

In addition to improving social perceptions, facial reanimation improves psychosocial health of patients with facial paralysis. Lindsay and colleagues[35] demonstrated that patients report significantly improved quality of life and FaCE scores after free gracilis muscle transfer. In addition, botulinum toxin treatment of facial synkinesis significantly improves patient quality of life.[36,37]

Considerations

The psychosocial implications of facial paralysis emerge from the influence on how patients interact with society. Notably, patients suffer from the loss of civil inattention, a disturbance in self-concept, and negative experiences with social interactions, resulting in lower quality of life. These consequences result from the multitude of aforementioned factors.

As described above, individuals interacting with patients with facial paralysis enter social interactions with a negative bias. The static facial deformity marked by asymmetry and the dynamic lack of expression pose significant obstacles to social well-being of patients.

Patient and provider education and understanding of the basic muscular and spatiotemporal facets of facial expressions and affect display are key to success. With this knowledge, providers should consider the following:

1. Restore dynamic function to the face whenever possible.
   - Prioritize reanimating the smile, as it forms the basis of positive affect display, positive

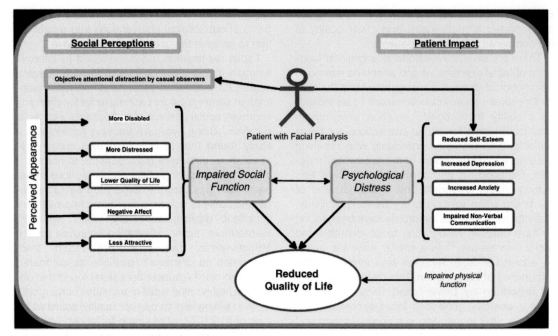

Fig. 1. Psychosocial impact of facial paralysis.

emotional experience, and a social cue for motivation of interpersonal interactions.

2. Reduce facial disfigurement
   - Improve facial symmetry, reconstruct facial contour deformities, reduce stigma of illness leading to paralysis (ie, inject the contralateral intact brow and corrugators, perform fat grafting, perform scar revision).
3. Improve attractiveness
   - Consider procedures that will enhance attractiveness in order to improve favorable inferences and first impressions of your patients (ie, facial and skin rejuvenation procedures).
4. Reduce negative facial cues
   - Work to reduce aspects of facial position that are inferred as negative (that is, elevate the ptotic brow surgically, treat the glabella with botulinum toxin in the corrugators, chemodenervate the platysma and depressor anguli oris in synkinetic patients, treat the buccinator in synkinesis, as it can signal irony and contempt when used with zygomaticus).
5. Address emotional well-being
   - Screen for depression and adjustment disorder in patients and refer for treatment if needed.
6. Train patients
   - Rehabilitate patients with the knowledge of social inferences (ie, train to reduce asymmetry in smile onset, practice to maximize dental show in the context of smile extent

and mouth angle, reduce constrained smiles, as they can be misinterpreted as contempt, educate on appropriate social cues with expected reciprocal facial movements).

SUMMARY

Facial paralysis has a significant psychosocial impact on patients (**Fig. 1**). Patients suffer from having negative observer perceptions, disruptions of self-perceptions, and impaired social interactions. As a consequence, patients have impaired social function, altered self-concept, psychological distress, and reduced quality of life. Fortunately, facial reanimation can help alleviate some of the psychosocial burden of facial paralysis. Nonetheless, treating physicians should be vigilant regarding identifying psychological distress and consider referral for evaluation and treatment if necessary.

CLINICS CARE POINTS

- Patients with facial paralysis are perceived as less attractive, having a more negative affect, and having a lower quality of life.

- Observers may potentially be unable to recognize facial expression in patients with facial paralysis, or erroneously interpret facial cues.

- Individuals with facial paralysis suffer from reduced self-esteem, increased anxiety, worse depression, and reduced quality of life.
- Facial reanimation improves the psychosocial morbidity of facial paralysis
- Early detection of mental health issues in patients with facial paralysis may improve overall care of this patient population.
- Think globally about facial function and consider additional treatments to improve facial inferences by observers, considering attractiveness and disfigurement.
- Train and educate patients about the observer perspective and social cues associated with facial movements.

DISCLOSURE

The authors have nothing to disclose.

REFERENCES

1. Frith C. Role of facial expressions in social interactions. Philosophical Trans R Soc Lond Ser B Biol Sci 2009;364(1535):3453–8.
2. Baaren RBV, Holland RW, Kawakami K, et al. Mimicry and prosocial behavior. Psychol Sci 2004; 15(1):71–4.
3. Shaw WC. Folklore surrounding facial deformity and the origins of facial prejudice. Br J Plast Surg 1981; 34(3):237–46.
4. Black JD, Girotto JA, Chapman KE, et al. When my child was born: cross-cultural reactions to the birth of a child with cleft lip and/or palate. Cleft Palate Craniofacial J 2009;46(5):545–8.
5. Ishii L, Dey J, Boahene KD, et al. The social distraction of facial paralysis: objective measurement of social attention using eye-tracking. Laryngoscope 2016;126(2):334–9.
6. Helwig NE, Sohre NE, Ruprecht MR, et al. Dynamic properties of successful smiles. PLoS One 2017; 12(6):e0179708.
7. Ishii LE, Godoy A, Encarnacion CO, et al. What faces reveal: impaired affect display in facial paralysis. Laryngoscope 2011;121(6):1138–43.
8. Bogart K, Tickle-Degnen L, Ambady N. Communicating without the face: holistic perception of emotions of people with facial paralysis. Basic Appl Soc Psychol 2014;36(4):309–20.
9. Ishii L, Godoy A, Encarnacion CO, et al. Not just another face in the crowd: society's perceptions of facial paralysis. Laryngoscope 2012;122(3):533–8.
10. Mun SJ, Park KT, Kim Y, et al. Characteristics of the perception for unilateral facial nerve palsy. Eur Arch Otorhinolaryngol 2015;272(11):3253–9.
11. Li MK, Niles N, Gore S, et al. Social perception of morbidity in facial nerve paralysis. Head & neck 2016;38(8):1158–63.
12. Goines JB, Ishii LE, Dey JK, et al. Association of facial paralysis-related disability with patient- and observer-perceived quality of life. JAMA Facial Plast Surg 2016;18(5):363–9.
13. Dey JK, Ishii LE, Nellis JC, et al. Comparing patient, casual observer, and expert perception of permanent unilateral facial paralysis. JAMA Facial Plast Surg 2017;19(6):476–83.
14. Ryzenman JM, Pensak ML, Tew JM Jr. Facial paralysis and surgical rehabilitation: a quality of life analysis in a cohort of 1,595 patients after acoustic neuroma surgery. Otology & neurotology: official publication of the American Otological Society, American Neurotology Society [and] European Academy of Otology and Neurotology 2005;26(3): 516–21. discussion 521.
15. Prats-Golczer VE, Gonzalez-Cardero E, Exposito-Tirado JA, et al. Impact of dysfunction of the facial nerve after superficial parotidectomy: a prospective study. Br J Oral Maxillofac Surg 2017;55(8): 798–802.
16. VanSwearingen JM, Cohn JF, Turnbull J, et al. Psychological distress: linking impairment with disability in facial neuromotor disorders. Otolaryngol Head Neck Surg 1998;118(6):790–6.
17. Saito DM, Cheung SW. A comparison of facial nerve disability between patients with Bell's palsy and vestibular schwannoma. J Clin Neurosci 2010; 17(9):1122–5.
18. Kleiss IJ, Hohman MH, Susarla SM, et al. Health-related quality of life in 794 patients with a peripheral facial palsy using the FaCE scale: a retrospective cohort study. Clin Otolaryngol 2015;40(6):651–6.
19. Leong SC, Lesser TH. A national survey of facial paralysis on the quality of life of patients with acoustic neuroma. Otol Neurotol 2015;36(3):503–9.
20. Nellis JC, Ishii M, Byrne PJ, et al. Association among facial paralysis, depression, and quality of life in facial plastic surgery patients. JAMA Facial Plast Surg 2017;19(3):190–6.
21. Strobel L, Renner G. Quality of life and adjustment in children and adolescents with Moebius syndrome: evidence for specific impairments in social functioning. Res Dev disabilities 2016;53-54: 178–88.
22. Fu L, Bundy C, Sadiq SA. Psychological distress in people with disfigurement from facial palsy. Eye (London) 2011;25(10):1322–6.
23. Bradbury ET, Simons W, Sanders R. Psychological and social factors in reconstructive surgery for hemi-facial palsy. J Plast Reconstr Aesthet Surg 2006;59(3):272–8.
24. Walker DT, Hallam MJ, Ni Mhurchadha S, et al. The psychosocial impact of facial palsy: our experience

in one hundred and twenty six patients. Clin Otolaryngol 2012;37(6):474–7.

25. Kim MJ, Neta M, Davis FC, et al. Botulinum toxin-induced facial muscle paralysis affects amygdala responses to the perception of emotional expressions: preliminary findings from an A-B-A design. Biol Mood Anxiety Disord 2014;4:11.

26. Bate S, Cook SJ, Mole J, et al. First report of generalized face processing difficulties in mobius sequence. PloS One 2013;8(4):e62656.

27. Lewis MB. Exploring the positive and negative implications of facial feedback. Emotion (Washington, DC) 2012;12(4):852–9.

28. Ekman P. Facial expression and emotion. Am Psychol 1993;48:384–92.

29. Korb S, Wood A, Banks CA, et al. Asymmetry of facial mimicry and emotion perception in patients with unilateral facial paralysis. JAMA Facial Plast Surg 2016;18(3):222–7.

30. Lyford-Pike S, Helwig NE, Sohre NE, et al. Predicting perceived disfigurement from facial function in patients with unilateral paralysis. Plast Reconstr Surg 2018;142(5):722e–8e.

31. Dey JK, Ishii LE, Byrne PJ, et al. Seeing is believing: objectively evaluating the impact of facial reanimation surgery on social perception. Laryngoscope 2014;124(11):2489–97.

32. Dey JK, Ishii M, Boahene KD, et al. Facial reanimation surgery restores affect display. Otol Neurotol 2014;35(1):182–7.

33. Dey JK, Ishii M, Boahene KD, et al. Changing perception: facial reanimation surgery improves attractiveness and decreases negative facial perception. Laryngoscope 2014;124(1):84–90.

34. Su P, Ishii LE, Joseph A, et al. Societal value of surgery for facial reanimation. JAMA Facial Plast Surg 2017;19(2):139–46.

35. Lindsay RW, Bhama P, Hadlock TA. Quality-of-life improvement after free gracilis muscle transfer for smile restoration in patients with facial paralysis. JAMA Facial Plast Surg 2014;16(6):419–24.

36. Mehta RP, Hadlock TA. Botulinum toxin and quality of life in patients with facial paralysis. Arch Facial Plast Surg 2008;10(2):84–7.

37. Streitova H, Bares M. Long-term therapy of benign essential blepharospasm and facial hemispasm with botulinum toxin A: retrospective assessment of the clinical and quality of life impact in patients treated for more than 15 years. Acta Neurol Belg 2014;114(4):285–91.

Static Sling Options for Facial Paralysis
Now Versus 10 Years Ago

Almoaidbellah Rammal, MD[a,b], John Yoo, MD[a], Damir Matic, MD[c],*

KEYWORDS

- Facial nerve paralysis • Static reanimation • Facial reanimation

KEY POINTS

- The main goal of static reanimation is to restore symmetry at rest.
- Palmaris or plantaris tendon graft static suspension provides long lasting results compared to other static suspension materials.
- Treatment of levator palpebrae superioris hyperactivity should be done through tightening and elevating the lower eyelid rather than placing a heavier upper eyelid weight.
- Brow lift and eyelid weight procedures should not be done at the same time.
- Addressing both upper and lower eyelid laxity is important to treat excessive tearing.

INTRODUCTION

Facial paralysis has devastating consequences emotionally, aesthetically, and functionally.[1,2] Facial reanimation treatments are broadly divided into reinnervation, static, and dynamic. Static procedures can provide symmetry at rest and the illusion of facial tone but do not offer movement. These procedures do not provide symmetry during function.[3]

Facial paralysis management needs to be considered based on location and degree of functional loss. It may involve the entire face or different anatomic units, such as the brow, upper eyelid, lower eyelid, midface, and lower lip. Paralysis is either complete or partial loss of function and it is reversible or irreversible based on the cause of nerve/muscle injury.[4] Paralysis is generally considered irreversible if present for longer than 2 years or when the distal nerve/motor unit is not present.[5]

Among the goals of restoration for the irreversibly paralyzed face is to achieve symmetry and improve static function, such as oral competence in repose. This involves static suspension of the oral commissure and lateral ala to recreate a nasolabial fold. In this article we focus on the static approaches for facial reanimation.[3]

Many static procedures have been described to treat the paralyzed face. Choosing the best option depends on patient factors, such as age and comorbidities, and injury factors, such as duration, location, and prognosis.[5] The approaches for static suspension also depend on whether the procedures will be performed at the time of ablative surgery or as a secondary procedure.

Table 1 summarizes the static reanimation procedures discussed in this article.

MATERIAL

A variety of materials have been used during static procedures including suspension sutures; alloplastic materials (eg, Gore-Tex); acellular dermal matrix; and native tissues, such as fascia or tendon grafts.[6,7]

[a] Department of Otolaryngology – Head and Neck Surgery, Western University, Victoria Hospital, London Health Science Centre, 800 Commissioners Road East, Room B3-429, London, ON N6A 5W9, Canada;
[b] Department of Otolaryngology – Head and Neck Surgery, King Abdul-Aziz University, Jeddah, Saudi Arabia;
[c] Division of Plastic and Reconstructive Surgery, Department of Surgery, Schulich School of Medicine and Dentistry, University of Western Ontario, Victoria Hospital, 800 Commissioners Road East, PO Box 5010, London, ON N6A 5W9, Canada
* Corresponding author.
E-mail address: Damir.Matic@lhsc.on.ca

Facial Plast Surg Clin N Am 29 (2021) 375–381
https://doi.org/10.1016/j.fsc.2021.03.010

Table 1
Summary of static reanimation procedures

Region	Technique
Brow	Direct brow lift
Upper eyelid	Eyelid weight Lateral tarsorrhaphy
Lower eyelid	Lateral strip canthopexy Lower eyelid suspension with tendon
Nasal base	Alar base suspension
Midface	Nasolabial fold suspension
Mouth	Oral commissure suspension
Upper/lower lip	Tendon suspension

The palmaris or plantaris tendons have become our preferred material because of their tendency to resist laxity and maintain their position over time. These tendons are easily harvested at the time of ablative surgery and have the benefits of being native tissue. The palmaris tendon is easily identified on clinical examination. In patients who are missing this tendon, other options include plantaris or the long extensors of the toes (third or fourth). Note that the plantaris longus tendon may also be absent in some patients.

For midface resuspension, a longer tendon is often required. As a result, the plantaris longus is the preferred option. Preoperative MRI or intraoperative exploration is performed to identify the tendon.

Advantages of using tendon grafts include: resistance to lengthening, lower relapse rate, very long sling (eg, plantaris longus), and minimal to no donor deficit. However, a separate donor site scar is required.

EYE COMPLEX STATIC PROCEDURES

The immediate priority in managing a patient with facial paralysis is ensuring adequate corneal protection. This is important regardless of whether or not the paralysis is reversible. The eye complex is considered in three segments that include the brow, upper lid, and lower lid.

Brow ptosis can cause a reduction in the visual field and asymmetry and upper eyelid paralysis can lead to corneal dryness and exposure. This in turn can cause epiphora and pain and may lead to corneal ulceration.[3]

Lower eyelid paralysis results in poor tear film maintenance and drainage leading to epiphora. With time, this lower eyelid laxity results in scleral show and ultimately to ectropion further worsening corneal exposure, epiphora, and pain.

Excessive tearing is a common symptom that is bothersome for patients with facial paralysis. The causes of excessive tearing include: (1) corneal exposure, dryness, and irritation because of poor upper lid closure; (2) loss of lower lid support with the puncta falling away from the globe resulting in inefficiency in the canalicular system; and (3) loss of the pump action of the orbicularis oculi on the lacrimal sac affecting normal drainage.[3,8,9]

Improvement in upper eyelid closure may reduce symptoms of irritation and thereby excessive lacrimation. However, better upper lid function alone does not address the tear drainage system. Therefore, addressing the position and tone of the lower eyelid should be considered to reduce epiphora.

We consistently see an improvement in upper lid closure following lower lid tendon suspension. The exact mechanism of this finding is unclear but may be related to a transmission of tension laterally from the lower lid to the upper lid. As a result, we often stage the two procedures. Lower lid suspension and tightening is generally performed first followed by upper lid weight insertion. This approach has allowed us to downsize the weight needed for appropriate upper lid closure.

Direct Brow Lift

A brow lift may be indicated for aesthetic or functional deficits. Eyebrow ptosis may result in facial asymmetry or visual field impairment secondary to excess upper eyelid skin.

Direct brow lift, unlike other techniques, such as midforehead lift, coronal incision, and endoscopic brow lift, is simple, quick, and repeatable with immediate results. It can also be performed under local anesthetic. Especially in patients with irreversible paralysis, a direct brow excision provides the best long-term outcome with a lower rate of relapse. This procedure can also be combined with botulinum toxin injections on the contralateral side for added symmetry even during motion. The one disadvantage to this approach is an external scar just above the brow, which is more visible in younger patients or those with less brow hair **Fig. 1**.

This procedure should be performed with caution when performed simultaneously with an upper eyelid procedure, such as weight insertion or blepharoplasty, because brow elevation can reduce eyelid closure.

Upper Eyelid Weight

Upper lid weight insertion is indicated in patients with symptomatic incomplete upper eyelid closure

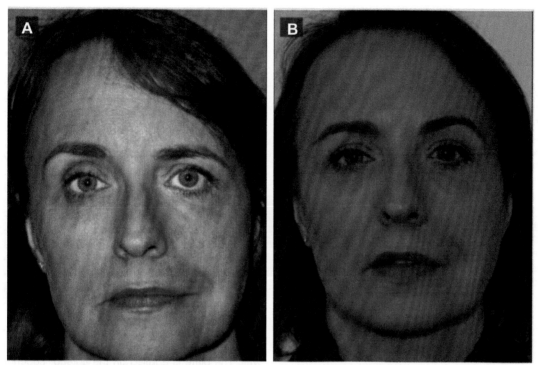

Fig. 1. Direct brow lift. (*A*) Preoperative picture showing irreversible brow ptosis. (*B*) Six months postoperative picture showing symmetric brow position at rest.

and provides a significant reduction in lagophthalmos and improvement in corneal coverage.[10] Upper lid loading with either a gold or platinum weight as a static procedure is simple, safe, effective, and reversible. Compared with gold, platinum weights have a thinner profile and cause less foreign body reaction, which can improve esthetics and lower the risk of extrusion; however, they are more expensive.[11]

Some patients over time can develop hyperactivity of the levator palpebrae superioris muscle. These patients often present with progressively poorer upper lid closure despite weight insertion. We have found that lid closure is most effectively improved in these patients by lower lid tightening and suspension rather than replacing an existing weight with a heavier one.

Lateral Tarsorrhaphy

Lateral tarsorrhaphy is a simple and reversible procedure that is done under local anesthetic. Indications include: a temporary measure to protect the cornea while awaiting a definitive procedure to improve eyelid function, an emergency measure when there is the possibility of imminent visual loss caused by exposure, in combination with other eyelid procedures, or as a salvage procedure when other treatments have failed. Early

intervention should be considered especially in patients with a poor or absent Bell phenomenon.

LOWER EYELID
Lateral Strip Canthopexy

Lateral strip canthopexy is another static reanimation option for patients with mild to moderate lower lid laxity. These patients often present with scleral show or mild ectropion. This procedure only tightens the lateral two-thirds of the lid (lateral to the medial limbus) and therefore does not address any medial laxity. It is performed in isolation or in combination with a lower lid sling procedure if lid shortening is also necessary.

Lower Eyelid Suspension: Tendon Sling

Lower eyelid suspension with tendon sling is our preferred procedure for patients with moderate to severe ectropion. Unlike a lateral strip canthopexy, the tendon sling addresses medial and lateral lower lid laxity and can also tighten and further suspend the medial canthal tendon. Young patients with mild lid laxity, patients with relative proptosis (positive vector), or malar hypoplasia are relative contraindications for this procedure. Specifically, patients with a negative vector can have the lid/sling migrate inferiorly under the globe worsening lid position so great care should be taken in this patient population.

Approach

A modified blepharoplasty incision (15–20 mm) within the medial aspect of the supratarsal fold is performed through the orbicularis muscle. Medial traction allows access to the periosteum of the nasofrontal junction and medial orbital wall, which is then incised and lifted. This allows exposure of the medial orbital wall, nasofrontal junction, and supraorbital rim.

A lateral canthotomy incision is performed to access the lateral orbital wall. The periosteum of the lateral orbital rim is incised and elevated allowing exposure of the lateral orbital rim and internal lateral orbit. In cases when the lower lid is also lax, a lateral tarsal strip procedure can also be performed, which allows shortening of the lid by 5 to 8 mm.

Once harvested, the tendon is split using a scalpel into a 1- to 2-mm-thick strip. The harvested mini tendon is threaded along the ciliary margin of the lower lid using a Keith needle. The needle is prebent to better follow the gentle curve of the eyelid. The needle is brought out of the skin just lateral to the inferior punctum. The needle is reinserted through the same puncture site, allowing a change in direction. It is passed either through the medial canthal tendon, or deep to it avoiding the canalicular system (**Figs. 2** and **3**).

Lateral fixation of the tendon sling is done by drilling a hole, using a 2.0-mm drill, through the lateral orbital wall just below the frontozygomatic suture. The hole within the lateral orbit is placed 8 to 10 mm posterior to the orbital rim. Laterally, the tendon is passed through the hole previously drilled in the lateral wall from medial to lateral. The tendon is looped and secured to itself using a 3–0 nonresorbable suture.

Medially, the end of the tendon is oversewn using a 3–0 nonresorbable suture to allow for sufficient purchase of the fixation wire. The suture is passed multiple times through the tendon to sufficiently grab the tissue of the tendon. A 28- or 30-gauge stainless steel wire is passed through the suture, holding the tendon indirectly without risking pull through.

A plate is adapted to the anatomy of the anterior superior part of the medial orbital rim and medial wall. The plate is applied on the anterior superior part of the medial orbital rim.

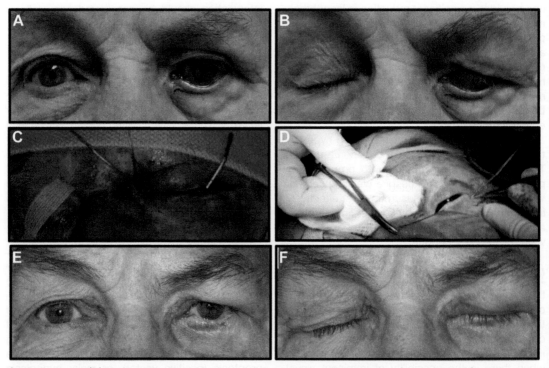

Fig. 2. Lower eyelid static suspension technique. (*A*) Preoperative photographs of a patient with severe ectropion. (*B*) Preoperative attempting eyes closure. (*C*) Intraoperative depiction of tendon position. (*D*) Tendon is threaded along the ciliary margin of the lower lid using a Keith needle. (*E*) Postoperative resting position after lower eyelid tendon suspension and upper eyelid gold weight insertion. (*F*) Postoperative eyes closed.

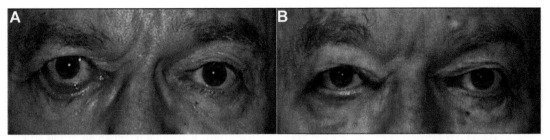

Fig. 3. Transnasal lower lid tendon suspension with gold weight implant and direct brow lift. (*A*) Patient with irreversible facial paralysis of the right side presenting with a painful, dry eye caused by loss of eyelid closure, lower lid ectropion, and brow ptosis. (*B*) Eight years postoperative result.

The tendon is placed superior and posterior to the lacrimal crest. Then the tendon is fixed medially by passing the holding wire through the most posterior hole of the plate. The tendon sling, once positioned, tightens the medial canthal tendon, the medial lower eyelid, and addresses the medial ectropion. Final tightening of the tendon sling is now performed.

Once satisfactory lower lid position and tension has been achieved, the wire is twisted and tightened over one of the screws used to fixate the plate to the frontal bone or onto a separate screw.

Alternatively, the medial tendon is secured transnasally forgoing the need for plate fixation. This technique can offer longer term stability of the tendon reducing the risk of the wire, suture, or tendon tearing on the medial orbital wall plate. However, this technique is more technically challenging, and a contralateral upper lid incision is needed.[9]

Another option for medial tendon fixation includes wrapping the tendon around and suturing it to the medial canthus without any bone fixation. Although this technique is technically easier, it does not adequately address medial lid and canthal laxity and often results in ongoing medial globe exposure.

Finally, if a lateral strip canthopexy is also performed, it is now completed. Otherwise a layered closure of the cantholysis is completed.

Antibiotic drops are provided 3 to 5 days postoperatively. It is important to maintain lubrication and protection of the eye. Physical protection through eyewear may be necessary depending on occupation and environmental conditions.

A more detailed description of the lower lid sling procedure is found at https://surgeryreference. aofoundation.org/cmf/reconstruction/facial-nerve.

MIDFACE AND MOUTH

The consequences of midface paralysis are nasal airway obstruction (external and internal nasal valve collapse), asymmetric smile, loss of oral competence, and speech difficulty. The goal is to achieve symmetry of the lower face only at repose. This involves static suspension of the oral commissure and lateral ala to recreate a nasolabial fold.[4]

Static Suspension of the Nasal Ala

A thin strip of palmaris/plantaris tendon is used to suspend and lateralize the nasal ala. This is performed through an alar crease incision in the nasal vestibule. The tendon is wrapped around the subcutaneous tissue of the alar base and fixated to itself with nonresorbable sutures. Laterally, the tendon is fixated with sutures to the deep temporal fascia through a temporal incision.

STATIC SUSPENSION OF THE ORAL COMMISSURE WITH TENDONS

In primary reconstruction, the existing surgical exposure (often a parotidectomy-type incision) is used to place the tendon slings into position. In secondary reconstruction, a temporal hairline and nasolabial fold incision are required. It is beneficial to mark the position of the new nasolabial fold and the desired vector of pull with the patient in a sitting position before general anesthesia.

In secondary reconstruction, the tendon is tunneled from the temporal incision to the fixation points around the mouth. This allows positioning the tendon in a similar vector of pull as the zygomaticus major muscle.

Separate tunnels are created at the level of nasolabial fold. The tendon is woven back and forth through them to achieve multiple points of fixation, recreating the nasolabial fold and suspending the commissure (**Fig. 4**). Typically, the orbicularis oris at the modiolus is suspended to the most distal aspect of the zygomatic arch or malar eminence, and the remaining points of fixation that create the upper nasolabial fold are anchored to the adjacent deep temporal fascia using permanent sutures. Slight overcorrection is

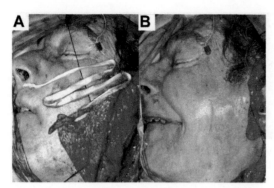

Fig. 4. Static suspension after resection of midfacial facial nerve branches. (*A*) Location of plantaris longus tendon demonstrated. (*B*) In situ placement depicting the pulling vector.

often necessary, because over time, with ongoing perioperative edema, some loosening occurs.

Postoperatively, patients are kept on a soft, nonchew diet for 2 to 3 weeks and are asked to

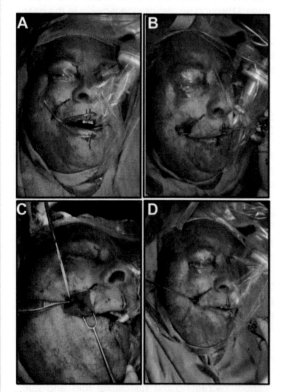

Fig. 5. Lower and upper lip static suspension using palmaris tendon. (*A*) Intraoperative location of palmaris tendon graft showing the two thin strips created by splitting the distal end of the tendon. (*B*) Tendon anchored laterally through a nasolabial incision. (*C, D*) The tendon strips are threaded along the substance of the muscular red lip and anchored medially (just past midline) using a permeant suture.

minimize their exertion to reduce the risk of inadvertent suspension release.

LOWER LIP

The signs and symptoms of lower lip paralysis include asymmetry during speech, loss of oral competence, inadvertent lip biting, and speech difficulty.

Excessive horizontal lengthening of the lip can occur with long-standing paralysis and unopposed contralateral pull. Because of atrophy of the orbicularis muscle, the red lip can thin and lengthen.

Horizontal Shortening of the Lower Lip

In cases of prolonged irreversible paralysis of the lower lip, horizontal shortening of the lower lip is a simple procedure that can improve symmetry at rest, oral competence, speech, and cosmesis. Patients should be aware of the possible need to repeat this procedure over time because of continued unopposed pull from the contralateral side. This procedure should be avoided when muscle recovery is expected. In addition, botulinum toxin injections in the contralateral depressor muscles can improve symmetry at rest and during function, further improving oral competence and speech in some patients.

Static Suspension of the Lower and Upper Lip

Using the same palmaris or plantaris tendon used for the oral commissure suspension, two thin strips are created by splitting the distal end of the tendon. These strips are then tunneled and attached to the upper and the lower lip (just past midline) using a permanent suture. The tendon strips are threaded along the substance of the muscular red lip and anchored medially within the lip substance and laterally to the commissure. Positioning the tendons in this manner maintains the length of the lip over time and may reduce the need for a lip-shortening procedure in the future (**Fig. 5**).

ANCILLARY PROCEDURES

As a result of long-lasting flaccid paralysis, the muscles of facial-expression atrophy. This leads to ptosis of the muscles, their attachments, and of the overlying soft tissue. Procedures, such as rhytidectomy of the face and neck, help tighten the ptotic soft tissues and can improve the efficacy of static sling procedures. Superficial Muscular Aponeurotic System (SMAS) plication and deep plane facelifts have been shown to improve the final result of the static procedures and patient satisfaction.[12] Note that these ancillary procedures should be performed as a final stage after other static procedures.

SUMMARY

Static suspension procedures provide immediate results, improved resting position, and may be useful to augment other techniques. At our center, tendon graft static suspensions are commonly used as sole treatments in elderly patients, patients with poor oncologic prognoses, or as adjunctive to other procedures to support the resting position.

CLINICS CARE POINTS

- Damage to the eye is the most serious functional injury that can result from facial nerve paralysis.

- Palmaris or plantaris tendon graft static suspensions provide longer lasting results compared with other static suspension materials and have the benefit of being autologous.

- Addressing upper and lower eyelid laxity is important in achieving efficient lid closure, corneal protection, and for treating excessive tearing.

- Treatment of levator palpebrae superioris hyperactivity should be done through tightening lower eyelid procedures, not by placing a heavier eyelid weight.

- Brow lift and upper eyelid weight procedures should not be done at the same time.

DISCLOSURE

The authors have nothing to disclose.

REFERENCES

1. Ishii L, Godoy A, Encarnacion CO, et al. Not just another face in the crowd: society's perceptions of facial paralysis. Laryngoscope 2012;122(3):533–8.
2. Faris C, Lindsay R. Current thoughts and developments in facial nerve reanimation. Curr Opin Otolaryngol Head Neck Surg 2013;21(4):346–52.
3. Sahovaler A, Yeh D, Yoo J. Primary facial reanimation in head and neck cancer. Oral Oncol 2017;74:171–80.
4. Jowett N, Hadlock TA. An evidence-based approach to facial reanimation. Facial Plast Surg Clin North Am 2015;23(3):313–34.
5. Lafer MP, Teresa MO. Management of long-standing flaccid facial palsy: static approaches to the brow, midface, and lower lip. Otolaryngol Clin North Am 2018;51(6):1141–50.
6. Jowett N, Hadlock TA. A contemporary approach to facial reanimation. JAMA Facial Plast Surg 2015;17(4):293–300.
7. Langille M, Singh P. Static facial slings: approaches to rehabilitation of the paralyzed face. Facial Plast Surg Clin North Am 2016;24(1):29–35.
8. Bhama P, Bhrany AD. Ocular protection in facial paralysis. Curr Opin Otolaryngol Head Neck Surg 2013;21(4):353–7.
9. Yoo J, Matic D. Transnasal tendon suspension for the paralyzed lower eyelid. J Plast Reconstr Aesthet Surg 2015;68(8):1072–8.
10. Chepeha DB, Yoo J, Birt C, et al. Prospective evaluation of eyelid function with gold weight implant and lower eyelid shortening for facial paralysis. Arch Otolaryngol Head Neck Surg 2001;127(3):299–303.
11. Silver AL, Lindsay RW, Cheney ML, et al. Thin-profile platinum eyelid weighting: a superior option in the paralyzed eye. Plast Reconstr Surg 2009;123(6):1697–703.
12. Biglioli F, Frigerio A, Autelitano L, et al. Deep-planes lift associated with free flap surgery for facial reanimation. J Craniomaxillofac Surg 2011;39(7):475–81.

Temporalis Tendon Transfer Versus Gracilis Free Muscle Transfer
When and Why?

G. Nina Lu, MD[a],*, Patrick J. Byrne, MD, MBA[b]

KEYWORDS

- Facial paralysis • Temporalis tendon transfer • Gracilis free tissue transfer

KEY POINTS

- Temporalis tendon transfers (T3) involve a single-stage outpatient procedure resulting in immediate improvement in resting tone and a volitional smile. Patients are unable to achieve true spontaneity and surgeons have less control over smile vector and shape.
- Modifications of the T3 with minimal incisional access, increased tendon harvest along the medial ramus, and intraoperative assessment of muscle tension relationship improves outcomes in this technique.
- Gracilis free muscle transfer (GFMT) allows a spontaneous smile, customized vectors, and greater excursion but requires longer surgical and recovery time, a delay before movement, and specialized equipment.
- Degree of resting symmetry is a key factor in surgical decision making between T3 and GFMT.

INTRODUCTION

Facial paralysis causes debilitating physical and psychological effects. The restriction of emotional expression, disruption of oral competence during speech and swallow, and static asymmetry cause significant impacts to quality of life and psychological distress.[1-4] Rehabilitation of lower facial movement, and specifically smile restoration, is a central focus of facial reanimation. Surgical treatments have documented improvements in quality of life, facial attractiveness, and psychosocial function.[5,6] Reinnervating native facial musculature is the preferred method of treatment when feasible.[7] No single muscle transfer option can duplicate the nuanced movements of mimetic facial musculature. The ideal technique would reestablish symmetry at rest and during smile. In patients with prolonged denervation, absence or myopathy of native facial musculature, abnormality of distal facial nerve branches, and/or incomplete paralysis with insufficient commissure movement, muscle transfer techniques are preferred for static and dynamic smile restoration. Although a myriad of muscle transfer techniques exists, the 2 most widely used techniques are the temporalis tendon transfer (T3) and gracilis free muscle transfer (GFMT). This article discusses surgical decision making between these 2 surgical options.

TEMPORALIS TENDON TRANSFER

Many variations using the temporalis muscle for facial reanimation exist. Gillies[8] initially described transposing the temporalis muscle belly over the zygomatic arch to suspend the paralyzed lip with a fascia lata extension in 1934. This technique

a Department of Otolaryngology, Division of Facial Plastic and Reconstructive Surgery, University of Washington, 325 9th Avenue, 4 West Clinic, Seattle, WA 98104, USA; b Head and Neck Institute, Cleveland Clinic Foundation, 9500 Euclid Avenue A71, Cleveland, OH 44106, USA
* Corresponding author.
E-mail address: ninalu@uw.edu

Facial Plast Surg Clin N Am 29 (2021) 383–388
https://doi.org/10.1016/j.fsc.2021.03.002
1064-7406/21/Published by Elsevier Inc.

causes a visible bulge over the zygoma accentuated by an adjacent hollow in the temporal donor site.[9] In addition, folding the muscle belly over the zygomatic arch alters the vector and dynamics of contraction and likely decreases contractile capacity. Improving on the donor site deformity and oral commissure excursion, McLaughlin[10] described an orthodromic use of the temporalis muscle via a coronoidectomy with fascia lata extension in 1949. Labbe and Huault[11] subsequently described the lengthening temporalis myoplasty (LTM), eliminating the need for a fascia graft extension by releasing the periosteal attachments of the posterior third of the temporalis muscle within the temporal fossa to create additional length.[11–13] Additional modifications of the orthodromic temporalis tendon transfer reduce and refine the use of fascia lata extension and use minimal access incisions.[14–17]

Orthodromic temporalis tendon transfer techniques and modifications are well described in the literature. Critical to maximizing contractility and commissure excursion, the temporalis muscle tension must be maintained as close to its optimal passive length as possible. Intraoperative muscle stimulation allows surgeons to objectively determine optimal muscle tension length.[17,18] Although classically described as inserting on the coronoid process, the temporalis tendon extends down the medial aspect of the mandibular ramus along the buccinator ridge as far as the mandibular third molar.[15] Additional length may be gained by dissecting along the medial aspect of the ramus and dividing the tendon as low as possible. In many patients, this modification obviates a fascia lata extension. Eliminating an adynamic segment and additional point of suture fixation reduces the risk of tendon dehiscence and improves the efficiency of commissure excursion. This dissection may be accomplished via a small nasolabial or intraoral incision. Objective outcomes of minimally invasive temporalis tendon transposition (MIT3) reveal distinct improvement in vertical commissure symmetry with smile and expert-graded Terzis score.[19] The authors prefer this MIT3 and comparative discussion in this article is based on this technique.[15]

Key advantages to this technique include:

1. A single-stage surgery that is routinely performed in the outpatient setting.
2. There is an immediate and reliable improvement in resting symmetry after surgery.
3. Volitional movement may begin immediately after surgery, although the authors suggest patients adhere to a soft diet and avoid volitional

movement for 6 weeks postoperatively to prevent tendon disinsertion or dehiscence from the commissure.
4. Minimal access incision via the nasolabial fold or oral mucosa may be used.
5. Pterygoid muscles compensate for temporalis muscle function, leading to minimal donor site morbidity.
6. Use of T3 does not preclude patients from receiving subsequent reanimation procedures such as GFMT.

Limitations of this technique include:

1. There is a fixed, single vector for oral commissure insertion. This limitation may be modified to some degree with variations in fascia lata extension grafts along the upper and lower lip.
2. Given the trigeminally mediated activation of the temporalis muscle, true spontaneity is unable to be achieved.
3. Although harvesting temporalis tendon along the medial ramus allows for increased tendon length, the quality of this distal tendon extension varies. Additional length may be required via fascia lata extension grafts or disinsertion of periosteal attachments within the temporal fossa or along the zygomatic arch.
4. Degree of commissure excursion achieved remains inconsistent. Excellent excursion may be achieved but this is likely to depend on preservation of native muscle tension, degree of insertion site dehiscence, and use of adynamic grafts.
5. A functioning temporalis muscle unit is required.
6. Neuromuscular retraining is necessary to optimize results.

GRACILIS FREE MUSCLE TRANSFER

The gracilis flap in smile reanimation was initially described by Harii and colleagues[9] in 1976 and has become the preferred technique in most institutions. Refinement of size of the gracilis muscle based on fascicular units allows increased precision in muscle size and tissue bulk transplanted.[20] Although the gracilis muscle has a single motor nerve, it comprises multiple nerve fascicles producing contraction in different regions of the muscle. Understanding gracilis neural fascicular anatomy has led to innovations such as the multivector gracilis in pursuit of a genuine enjoyment smile or Duchenne smile.[21] Duchenne smiles are characterized by periocular muscle activation with maximal dental display and high cheek elevation naturally associated with positive emotion.[22] In contrast, a social or Mona Lisa smile is a smile elicited mainly from the corners of the mouth with minimal dental display. By dividing the gracilis muscle into 3 functional neuromuscular units, separate muscle segments may be used to imitate levator labii superioris and orbicularis oculi activity in addition to zygomaticus activity. A slip of muscle placed medially and oriented slightly more vertically mimics levator labii superioris and a short slip of muscle placed within the lateral lower eyelid mimics orbicularis oculi activity. A wide variety of choices for neural innervation of GFMT exist. In the original description by Harii and colleagues,[9] the deep temporal nerve was used. Recognizing the need for facial nucleus input to achieve spontaneous movement, O'Brien and colleagues[23] described a 2-stage approach to innervate the gracilis muscle with a cross-facial nerve graft (CFNG). Because of the long distance (and consequently time) required for nerve regrowth, a CFNG is placed in a first-stage surgery and at least 4 months are allowed to elapse before muscle transplant. Although described innervation sources include spinal accessory, phrenic, and hypoglossal nerves, the masseteric nerve has become favored for its high axonal density, improved excursion, minimal donor site morbidity, and favorable proximity.[12] The ipsilateral facial nerve is the ideal donor nerve when feasible but is not available in most scenarios. Recent literature has supported using both a CFNG and the masseteric nerve for dual innervation of GFMT.[13] Although there are inadequate data to compare various methods of innervation, dual innervation is reported to be a safe procedure, movement initiation is similar to single masseteric nerve innervation, and most patients achieve spontaneity.[24]

Nuances of GFMT techniques vary between institution and no ideal technique has been established. Key advantages to GFMT include:

1. Spontaneous activation may be routinely achieved in GFMT with CFNG input.[25] Spontaneity is reported with trigeminal innervation, although this point is debated.[26]
2. Unencumbered adjustment of muscle size, position, and number of vectors allows approximation of a more natural smile based on patient characteristics.
3. Meaningful commissure excursion is reliably achieved in most patients.[27]
4. Adductor compensation for the gracilis muscle results in minimal morbidity in the donor site.
5. Multiple sources of neural input are available.

Limitations of this technique include:

1. Microvascular surgical expertise and equipment are needed to perform GFMT, and

patients require inpatient admission with free flap monitoring for 3 to 5 days postoperatively.
2. Patients require an initial procedure at least 4 months (and on average 6–9 months) before single-innervation GFMT with CFNG. Single-stage dual innervation with CFNG and masseter nerve has been described with satisfactory preliminary results.
3. Initiation of movement depends on neutral ingrowth. Movement starts around 4 to 6 months postoperatively and progresses over 2 to 3 years after surgery.
4. The addition of gracilis muscle may result in midfacial bulk requiring secondary revision.
5. Similar to T3, neuromuscular retraining is necessary to optimize results.

EVIDENCE-BASED OUTCOME COMPARISON

Few articles directly compare temporalis tendon transfer and GFMT outcomes. Existing studies use widely varied surgical techniques and heterogeneous outcome measures, limiting aggregate comparison.

Erni and colleagues[28] performed a comparison of 10 orthodromic T3s via the McLaughlin technique and a group of 7 heterogeneous muscle transfers (gracilis, latissimus dorsi, pectoralis minor) in 1999. They found no difference in resting symmetry outcomes between the 2 techniques but more excursion with free neuromuscular transfers (mean, 5.5 mm; standard deviation, 1.6 mm) versus T3 (1.7 mm, 0.8 mm). Observers rated overall aesthetic appearance of neuromuscular transfers as markedly impaired by cheek swelling and skin tethering.

Gousheh and Arasteh[29] retrospectively reviewed 505 2-stage, CFNG-innervated GFMTs with 73 antidromic temporalis muscle transpositions and 4 lengthening temporal myoplasties. Results were graded as excellent ($\geq$2 cm lateral commissure movement), good (1.5 to <2 cm), satisfactory (<1.5 cm), and failed (<1 cm). The gracilis group achieved 14% excellent, 76% good, 8% satisfactory, and 2% failed results, whereas the temporals muscle transfer achieved 30% good, 59% satisfactory, and 11% failed. LTM patients were all classified as satisfactory.

A systematic review from 2016 evaluated GFMT versus lengthening temporalis myoplasty and revealed no randomized and controlled clinical trials of these techniques and heterogeneity in objective measurements.[13] GFMT studies reported better commissure excursion compared with LTM studies, although few studies of LTM reported quantifiable data.

A retrospective study from the Netherlands compared 10 masseter-driven gracilis and 12 antidromic temporalis muscle transposition patients.[30] The investigators reviewed excursion measurements, Facial Clinimetric Evaluation (FaCE) scale scores, and casual observer ratings. Smile excursion and symmetry analysis via FACE-gram software showed no statistically significant differences. FaCE scale subscores differed by only 1.7 points in favor of GFMT and were not statistically different. Casual observer aesthetic assessment did not show a preference between the two techniques.

In 2018, Oyer and colleagues[31] performed a retrospective study evaluating patients with unilateral flaccid facial paralysis undergoing MIT3 (14 patients) versus GFMT (14 patients). They evaluated commissure position in vertical, horizontal, and angular dimensions in repose and with smile. Both groups had significant improvement in commissure symmetry in repose as well as with smile. The MIT3 group had increased improvement in angular symmetry compared with GFMT at rest and with smile. The GFMT group had improved vertical symmetry in repose and smile compared with the MIT3 group. Horizontal symmetry was most improved in the GFMT during smile and did not improve significantly in repose in either group. Commissure excursion was present in both groups with a larger improvement in the GFMT group (11.3 mm; 95% confidence interval [CI], 7.0–15.5 mm) versus the MIT3 group (4.8 mm; 95% CI, 0.2–9.3 mm). The GFMT group achieved commissure symmetry to within 1 mm of the contralateral side. Given the retrospective nature of this study, the investigators note a significantly older population receiving the MIT3 compared with the GFMT.

More recently, Nguyen and colleagues[32] retrospectively reviewed LTM (6 patients) with 2-stage CFNG GFMT (10 patients) in the pediatric population. LTM patients showed a significant increase in commissure excursion within 0 to 3 months postoperatively (3.33 ± 1.58 mm) with steady increase in excursion the first year after surgery up to 7.27 +/- 1.96 mm. GFMT patients showed movement at 3 to 6 months postoperatively (4.01 ± 1.77 mm) and, on average, 5.28 mm at more than 12 months postoperatively. Resting symmetry was improved in both groups with superolateral overcorrection noted in LTM patients.

PATIENT-CENTERED SURGICAL DECISION MAKING

Temporalis tendon transfers allow reliable, immediate improvement in static symmetry with a single-stage outpatient procedure. The MIT3 technique further reduces surgical dissection and the use of extension grafting. Dynamic outcomes can be excellent but are inconsistent. Based on the limited existing data, temporalis tendon transfers likely result in reduced commissure excursion compared with GFMT. Resting symmetry is at least equivalent and potentially superior to GFMT depending on the gracilis innervation source. GFMT has consistent dynamic excursion results, more tailored smile vectors, and the opportunity for spontaneous movement. These long-term benefits come at the upfront cost of a (likely) multi-staged, longer surgery with a protracted period before initiation of perceivable movement and the risk of midfacial bulk. Although morphologic change and asymmetry may occur with T3, this is typically related to nuances in insertion technique rather true facial bulk caused by the additional tissue.

Ultimately, surgeons aim to deliver the maximal psychological and functional benefit to their patients with the simplest, least morbid techniques. The larger change or improvement delivered to the patients, the more benefit they will likely receive. Resting symmetry is one definitive patient characteristic that demarcates the expected improvement achieved between the T3 and the GFMT. Simply put, the most consistent benefit achieved with T3 is improvement in resting symmetry. If a patient is relatively symmetric at rest, there is no opportunity to achieve a beneficial change in this aspect and the result depends on the dynamic movement (**Fig. 1**). Dynamic movement is more consistently achieved with GFMT. Thus, good resting symmetry diminishes temporalis tendon transfers from consideration. In cases of incomplete paralysis, GFMT is typically preferred to T3 for this reason. In contrast, if a patient has poor resting symmetry, a large beneficial change may be achieved from both gracilis or T3 and consideration turns to secondary factors described previously (**Fig. 2**). In these situations, the consideration for desired dynamic outcome, ability to tolerate a long anesthetic, life expectancy, and desire for immediate results comes into play.

The MIT3 technique is particularly advantageous for (1) medically complex patients who cannot undergo a prolonged anesthetic, and (2) patients with short or unclear prognosis who desire an immediate benefit. Surgeons should discuss with patients that MIT3 does not preclude future pursuit of GFMT if their prognoses or circumstances change. The GFMT best suits patients in good health and with the desire for the optimal smile outcome. Both techniques benefit

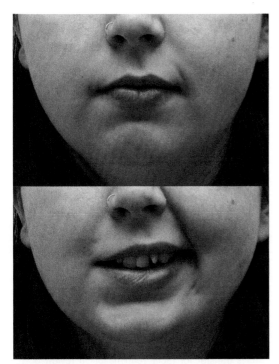

Fig. 1. Patient example of incomplete paralysis with good resting symmetry but weak dynamic movement.

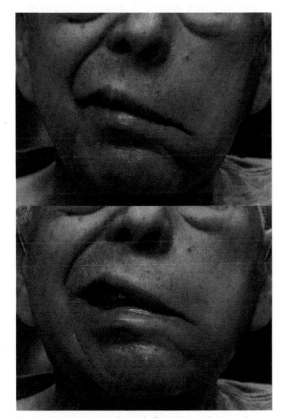

Fig. 2. Patient example with flaccid paralysis and poor resting symmetry and dynamic movement.

from facial neuromuscular retraining for optimal results. Shared decision making between the clinician and the patient should focus on the patient's goals and unique circumstances.

SUMMARY

The temporalis tendon transfer and GFMT are the 2 most used methods for smile rehabilitation in facial paralysis. Both techniques can achieve excellent outcomes. Patients may achieve the most natural, spontaneous smile outcomes with GFMT. Temporalis tendon transfer techniques consistently improve resting symmetry, allow immediate results, and involve a quicker recovery. Ultimately, surgical decision making should be centered on each patients' individual goals and situation.

DISCLOSURE

The authors have no commercial or financial conflicts of interest to disclose.

REFERENCES

1. Kleiss IJ, Hohman MH, Susarla SM, et al. Health-related quality of life in 794 patients with a peripheral facial palsy using the FaCE Scale: a retrospective cohort study. Clin Otolaryngol 2015;40(6):651–6.
2. Volk GF, Granitzka T, Kreysa H, et al. Nonmotor disabilities in patients with facial palsy measured by patient-reported outcome measures. Laryngoscope 2016;126(7):1516–23.
3. Ishii LE, Godoy A, Encarnacion CO, et al. What faces reveal: impaired affect display in facial paralysis. Laryngoscope 2011;121(6):1138–43.
4. VanSwearingen JM, Cohn JF, Turnbull J, et al. Psychological distress: linking impairment with disability in facial neuromotor disorders. Otolaryngol Head Neck Surg 1998;118(6):790–6.
5. Dey JK, Ishii M, Boahene KD, et al. Changing perception: facial reanimation surgery improves attractiveness and decreases negative facial perception. Laryngoscope 2014;124(1):84–90.
6. Lindsay RW, Bhama P, Hadlock TA. Quality-of-life improvement after free gracilis muscle transfer for smile restoration in patients with facial paralysis. JAMA Facial Plast Surg 2014;16(6):419–24.
7. Joseph AW, Kim JC. Management of flaccid facial paralysis of less than two years' duration. Otolaryngol Clin North Am 2018;51(6):1093–105.
8. Gillies H. Experiences with fascia lata grafts in the operative treatment of facial paralysis: (Section of Otology and Section of Laryngology). Proc R Soc Med 1934;27(10):1372–82.
9. Harii K, Ohmori K, Torii S. Free gracilis muscle transplantation, with microneurovascular anastomoses

for the treatment of facial paralysis. A preliminary report. Plast Reconstr Surg 1976;57(2):133–43.

10. McLaughlin CR. Surgical support in permanent facial paralysis. Plast Reconstr Surg (1946) 1953; 11(4):302–14.

11. Labbé D, Huault M. Lengthening temporalis myoplasty and lip reanimation. Plast Reconstr Surg 2000;105(4):1289–97 [discussion 1298].

12. Byrne PJ, Kim M, Boahene K, et al. Temporalis tendon transfer as part of a comprehensive approach to facial reanimation. Arch Facial Plast Surg 2007;9(4):234–41.

13. Boahene KD, Farrag TY, Ishii L, et al. Minimally invasive temporalis tendon transposition. Arch Facial Plast Surg 2011;13(1):8–13.

14. Croxson GR, Quinn MJ, Coulson SE. Temporalis muscle transfer for facial paralysis: a further refinement. Facial Plast Surg 2000;16(4):351–6.

15. Boahene KD, Ishii LE, Byrne PJ. In vivo excursion of the temporalis muscle-tendon unit using electrical stimulation: application in the design of smile restoration surgery following facial paralysis. JAMA Facial Plast Surg 2014;16(1):15–9.

16. Har-Shai Y, Gil T, Metanes I, et al. Intraoperative muscle electrical stimulation for accurate positioning of the temporalis muscle tendon during dynamic, one-stage lengthening temporalis myoplasty for facial and lip reanimation. Plast Reconstr Surg 2010;126(1):118–25.

17. Brichacek M, Sultan B, Boahene KD, et al. Objective outcomes of minimally invasive temporalis tendon transfer for prolonged complete facial paralysis. Plast Surg (Oakv) 2017;25(3):200–10.

18. Manktelow RT, Zuker RM. Muscle transplantation by fascicular territory. Plast Reconstr Surg 1984;73(5): 751–7.

19. Boahene KO, Owusu J, Ishii L, et al. The multivector gracilis free functional muscle flap for facial reanimation. JAMA Facial Plast Surg 2018;20(4):300–6.

20. Ekman P, Davidson RJ, Friesen WV. The Duchenne smile: emotional expression and brain physiology. II. J Personal Soc Psychol 1990;58(2):342–53.

21. O'Brien BM, Franklin JD, Morrison WA. Cross-facial nerve grafts and microneurovascular free muscle transfer for long established facial palsy. Br J Plast Surg 1980;33(2):202–15.

22. Roy M, Corkum JP, Shah PS, et al. Effectiveness and safety of the use of gracilis muscle for dynamic smile restoration in facial paralysis: a systematic review

and meta-analysis. J Plast Reconstr Aesthet Surg 2019;72(8):1254–64.

23. Bos R, Reddy SG, Mommaerts MY. Lengthening temporalis myoplasty versus free muscle transfer with the gracilis flap for long-standing facial paralysis: a systematic review of outcomes. J Craniomaxillofac Surg 2016;44(8):940–51.

24. Boonipat T, Robertson CE, Meaike JD, et al. Dual innervation of free gracilis muscle for facial reanimation: what we know so far. J Plast Reconstr Aesthet Surg 2020;73(12):2196–209.

25. Snyder-Warwick AK, Fattah AY, Zive L, et al. The degree of facial movement following microvascular muscle transfer in pediatric facial reanimation depends on donor motor nerve axonal density. Plast Reconstr Surg 2015;135(2):370e–81e.

26. Vila PM, Kallogjeri D, Yaeger LH, et al. Powering the gracilis for facial reanimation: a systematic review and meta-analysis of outcomes based on donor nerve. JAMA Otolaryngol Head Neck Surg 2020; 146(5):429–36.

27. Bhama PK, Weinberg JS, Lindsay RW, et al. Objective outcomes analysis following microvascular gracilis transfer for facial reanimation: a review of 10 years' experience. JAMA Facial Plast Surg 2014; 16(2):85–92.

28. Erni D, Lieger O, Banic A. Comparative objective and subjective analysis of temporalis tendon and microneurovascular transfer for facial reanimation. Br J Plast Surg 1999;52(3):167–72.

29. Gousheh J, Arasteh E. Treatment of facial paralysis: dynamic reanimation of spontaneous facial expression-apropos of 655 patients. Plast Reconstr Surg 2011;128(6):693e–703e.

30. van Veen MM, Dijkstra PU, le Coultre S, et al. Gracilis transplantation and temporalis transposition in long-standing facial palsy in adults: patient-reported and aesthetic outcomes. J Craniomaxillofac Surg 2018; 46(12):2144–9.

31. Oyer SL, Nellis J, Ishii LE, et al. Comparison of objective outcomes in dynamic lower facial reanimation with temporalis tendon and gracilis free muscle transfer. JAMA Otolaryngol Head Neck Surg 2018; 144(12):1162–8.

32. Nguyen PD, Faschan KS, Mazzaferro DM, et al. Comparison of lengthening temporalis myoplasty and free-gracilis muscle transfer for facial reanimation in children. J Craniofac Surg 2020;31(1):85–90.

Reinnervation with Selective Nerve Grafting from Multiple Donor Nerves

Shiayin F. Yang, MD[a], Jennifer C. Kim, MD[b],*

KEYWORDS

- Facial reanimation • Nerve substitution • Hypoglossal nerve transfer • Masseteric nerve transfer
- Cross-facial nerve grafting • Facial paralysis treatment

KEY POINTS

- This article reviews the different types of nerve substitution, their indications, and the pros and cons of each.
- The goal of nerve substitution is to restore dynamic and mimetic facial motion as well as resting facial tone and symmetry.
- Multiinnervation allows donor nerves to complement one another and avoid pitfalls inherent to individual donor nerves.

 Video content accompanies this article at http://www.facialplastic.theclinics.com.

INTRODUCTION

Nerve substitution is the preferred treatment of facial nerve injury when primary neurorrhaphy or cable grafting is not feasible. Nerve transfers are indicated when the proximal end of the facial nerve cannot be grafted but the distal nerve branches and facial muscles are viable. The ideal timing of neurotization surgery is within 2 years of facial nerve injury, as this has shown the most predictable results.[1]

Multiple cranial nerves have been used for nerve substitution; however, none can guarantee complete facial nerve recovery or restoration of normal facial function. The unpredictability of facial nerve outcomes lies in the complex nature of peripheral nerve regeneration and reinnervation. The ideal donor nerve depends on the type of nerve injury, time since injury, and patient factors. Nerve transfers can be used for direct motor neurotization, babysitter and double innervation techniques, and innervation of neuromuscular transplants. The most common nerve substitution procedures are discussed in this article.

NERVE SUBSTITUTION FOR TREATMENT OF FACIAL PARALYSIS
Hypoglossal-Facial Nerve Transfer

The hypoglossal-facial nerve transfer was first introduced in 1901 by Korte[2] and became widely popularized by Conley and Baker.[3] Initially, hypoglossal-facial nerve transfer involved complete transection of hypoglossal with end-to-end coaptation to the distal facial nerve. However, this resulted in unacceptable outcomes including functional deficits of speech, mastication, and swallowing, as well as hemifacial mass activation and synkinesis.

The procedure has since undergone multiple modifications to minimize morbidity. In 1991, May and colleagues[4] reported a technique of partial sacrifice of the hypoglossal nerve and end-to-side coaptation using an interposition graft. This

[a] Vanderbilt University Medical Center, 1215 21st Avenue South MCE, Suite 7209, Nashville, TN 37232, USA;
[b] University Michigan Health Systems, 1500 East Medical Center Drive, Ann Arbor, MI 48109, USA
* Corresponding author.
E-mail address: jennkim@med.umich.edu

Facial Plast Surg Clin N Am 29 (2021) 389–396
https://doi.org/10.1016/j.fsc.2021.03.003
1064-7406/21/© 2021 Elsevier Inc. All rights reserved.

technique maintained functional results while decreasing mass movement, synkinesis, and deficits of speech and mastication. Cusimano[5] reported longitudinal splitting of the hypoglossal nerve to preserve continuity to the tongue. Slattery and colleagues[6] described transposition of the intratemporal facial nerve with end-to-side coaptation, eliminating the need for an interposition graft.

Surgical technique

The senior author uses the technique of end-to-side coaptation with transposition of the intratemporal facial nerve. The procedure is performed through modified Blair parotidectomy incision. The main trunk of the facial nerve is identified using standard landmarks, and with assistance from an otology colleague, the facial nerve is transected at the geniculate ganglion and transposed inferiorly. The hypoglossal nerve is identified deep to the posterior belly of the digastric muscle and followed distally to the branching of the descendens hypoglossi. An incision is made in the hypoglossal nerve through 40% to 50% of its diameter, and the facial nerve is coapted end-to-side to the hypoglossal nerve. If extra length from the mastoid drill-out is not attainable, a cable graft using the greater auricular nerve may be used, although the senior author prefers direct coaptation by mobilizing the hypoglossal nerve superiorly with transection of the ansa if needed and performing direct coaptation very high proximally on the hypoglossal nerve at the level of transverse process of the second cervical spine. This avoids axonal loss from additional coaptation sites.

Advantages

- Large motor nerve with similar caliber to facial nerve
- Close proximity to facial nerve
- Restores facial tone
- Able to achieve voluntary smile with neuromuscular retraining

Disadvantages

- Unable to restore spontaneous mimetic function
- Neuromuscular retraining is necessary to simulate smile
- Potential for hemitongue atrophy, speech and mastication deficits, mass activation, and synkinesis with sacrifice of more than 50% of hypoglossal nerve

Masseteric-Facial Nerve Transfer

In 1978, Spira[7] introduced masseteric-facial nerve transfer for facial reanimation (**Fig. 1**). This procedure became a popular donor nerve due to its proximity, ease of dissection, length and caliber, minimal donor morbidity, and rapid functional recovery.[8] The masseteric nerve has more than 1500 axons,[9] which is a sufficient number to power the main trunk and produce reliable and powerful oral commissure excursion.[10] The masseteric nerve has also demonstrated significantly faster clinical recovery compared with the hypoglossal.[11]

The main critiques of this donor nerve are inability to recover mimetic function and poor facial tone in repose.[12,13] The absence of resting facial tone is most notable during speech, when the patient is unable to activate their masseter. Restoration of resting tone is important from both an aesthetic and a functional standpoint. Aesthetically, facial symmetry is only obtained with masseteric activation, whereas at rest there is obvious asymmetry between the 2 sides. From a functional standpoint, loss of facial tone has significant consequences for the eye and midface. Loss of orbicularis oculi tone and gravitational pull of the midface can cause paralytic ectropion, which can result in inadequate eyelid closure, exposure keratopathy, corneal ulceration, and blindness if not treated. Difficulties in mastication and speech are consequences of loss of buccinator tone. To

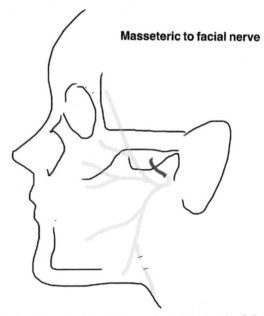

Masseteric to facial nerve

Fig. 1. Masseteric nerve transfer to the trunk of the facial nerve. Selective cervical branch neurectomy may be performed to reduce synkinesis involving the platysma.

address these shortfalls, the authors integrate static procedures with masseteric nerve transfer.[13]

Surgical technique

Through a preauricular incision, a cheek flap is elevated just over the parotidomasseteric fascia anterior to the anterior border of the masseter muscle. The parotid fascia is incised to identify buccal branches that are dissected retrograde. Facial nerve branches superior and inferior to the point of entry are identified and protected. Dissection can begin at a point 1 cm below the zygomatic arch and 3 cm anterior to the tragus.[14] Another approach to localize the nerve is the subzygomatic triangle, which is formed by the zygomatic arch, frontal branch of the facial nerve, and a perpendicular line through the temporomandibular joint.[15] The nerve travels along the deep part of the masseter muscle about 1.0 to 1.5 cm deep to the parotidomasseteric fascia. The nerve is traced distally and can be followed after it branches, including these branches in order to obtain as much length as possible (**Fig. 2**). The dissection is often bloody, which can make identification of the nerve difficult. Ways to identify the nerve if one is having difficulty is to use microcottonoids moistened with 1:1000 epinephrine to limit bleeding or to use nerve stimulator when in close proximity. Once the nerve is transected, it is coapted end-to-end to the main trunk or lower division of the facial nerve. Vein grafts are used to ensheath neurorrhaphies.

Advantages

- Large motor nerve with more than 1500 axons
- Close proximity to facial nerve facilitates direct coaptation
- Faster clinical recovery compared with hypoglossal nerve
- Minimal donor morbidity

Disadvantages

- Unable to restore spontaneous mimetic function
- Does not restore resting facial muscle tone
- Neuromuscular retraining is necessary to simulate smile

Masseteric-Facial, Cable Nerve Graft

Nerve substitution can also be used as an adjunct to facial nerve repair. Cable grafting of the facial nerve is performed when primary neurorrhaphy is not feasible. Expected recovery after cable grafting is about 6 to 12 months; however, this may vary depending on the preoperative facial nerve function. Owusu and colleagues[16] reported favorable outcomes with combining masseteric nerve transfer with facial nerve cable grafting (**Fig. 3**). They demonstrated fast return of oral commissure movement and decreased synkinesis. The addition of masseteric nerve transfer to cable grafting augments results through powering strong oral commissure excursion and providing neural input while awaiting nerve regeneration through the cable graft.

MULTIPLE NERVE SUBSTITUTIONS FOR TREATMENT OF FACIAL PARALYSIS
Masseteric-Facial, Hypoglossal-Facial Nerve Transfer

Dual innervation procedures are reanimation techniques that involve the use of donor nerve input from more than one cranial nerve. Each cranial

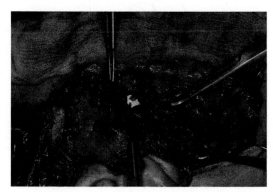

Fig. 2. Dissection to identify the masseteric nerve to be coapted to a buccal branch of facial nerve.

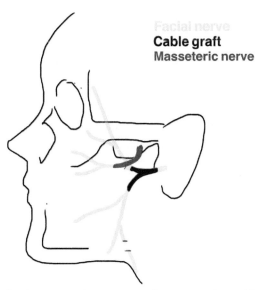

Facial nerve

Cable graft
Masseteric nerve

Fig. 3. Masseteric nerve transfer augmenting cable graft via coaptation to a buccal branch.

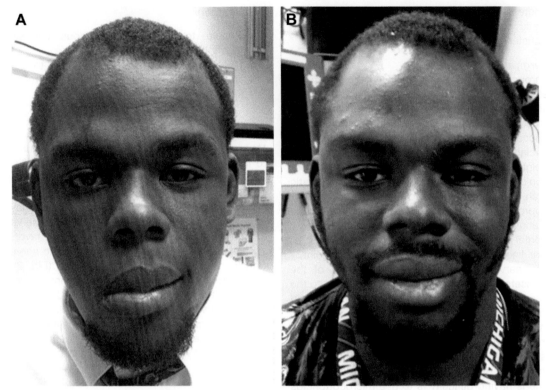

Fig. 4. (*A*) Preoperative photo of a patient with right facial nerve paralysis secondary to facial nerve hemangioma. (*B*) Postoperative photo, 9 months after dual innervation with hypoglossal and masseteric nerves.

nerve possesses inherent characteristics that influence its utility in facial reanimation. Dual innervation techniques leverage the inherent characteristics of different cranial nerves to complement one another and minimize the downfalls when an individual donor nerve is used on its own. The combination of the masseteric and hypoglossal nerves can be used to obtain good resting tone from the hypoglossal nerve and a more natural smile with clenching, as well as reduced synkinesis from the masseteric nerve (**Fig. 4**).

Surgical technique
Identification of the masseteric and hypoglossal nerves is performed as described earlier. The main trunk of the facial nerve is identified using standard landmarks, and, with assistance from an otology colleague, the facial nerve is transected at the geniculate ganglion and transposed inferiorly. An incision is made in the hypoglossal nerve through 50% of its diameter, and the facial nerve is coapted end-to-side to the hypoglossal. The masseteric nerve is coapted end-to-end to a large buccal branch (**Fig. 5**).

Advantages

- Voluntary smile with clenching from the masseteric nerve

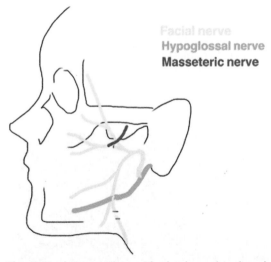

Facial nerve
Hypoglossal nerve
Masseteric nerve

Fig. 5. Dual innervation with the hypoglossal and masseteric nerves. The main trunk of the facial nerve is coapted end-to-side to the hypoglossal. The masseteric nerve is coapted to a buccal branch. Selective cervical branch neurectomy may be performed to reduce synkinesis involving the platysma.

- Recovery of resting facial tone from the hypoglossal nerve

Disadvantages

- Unable to restore spontaneous mimetic function
- Neuromuscular retraining is necessary to simulate smile
- Potential hemitongue atrophy, speech and mastication deficits, mass activation, and synkinesis with sacrifice of more than 40% of hypoglossal nerve

Masseteric-Facial, Hypoglossal-Facial Nerve Transfer, Cross-Face Nerve Graft

Inability to restore spontaneous, mimetic function is the main downfall of dual innervation with the masseteric and hypoglossal nerves. The only donor nerve that can provide spontaneous blink and emotive smile is the contralateral facial nerve; this can be used in facial reanimation by using an interposition graft to connect the affected side to the unaffected side, known as a cross-facial nerve graft (CFNG). CFNG is reliant on a long interposition nerve graft, which results in a significant delay from reanimation surgery to reinnervation of the target muscle. Thus, many surgeons combine CFNG with a babysitter nerve to allow for earlier reinnervation and preservation of the distal neuromuscular unit. Additional downfalls of CFNG include unpredictable outcomes and fewer donor axons compared with other donor nerves.[17] Adding CFNG with dual innervation by the hypoglossal and masseteric nerves allows for recovery of resting facial tone, smile, and mimetic midface and ocular function (**Fig. 6**). In addition, the intact side function is powered down, which improves overall symmetry.

Surgical technique

Masseteric and hypoglossal nerve transfers are performed as described earlier. The sural nerve is harvested from the lower extremity, which can be performed with or without the use of an endoscope. Through a facelift style preauricular incision on the unaffected side, a cheek flap is elevated and dissection carried anteriorly to the buccal fat pad. The facial nerve branch to the zygomaticus major may be identified at Zuker's point, which is located halfway along a line drawn between the root of the helix and the oral commissure.[18] The facial nerve branches can be traced in a retrograde fashion to identify a donor nerve of large caliber and axonal load. Using a nerve stimulator, the branch with the most specificity for activation of the zygomaticus major is identified and

transected. The CFNG is coapted end-to-end to the selected nerve, tunneled under the upper lip, and brought to the affected side where it is coapted to a zygomatic branch directing input to the midface and lower lid (**Fig. 7**).

Advantages

- Voluntary smile with clenching from the masseteric nerve
- Recovery of resting facial tone from the hypoglossal nerve
- Partial restoration of spontaneous, mimetic function from CFNG

Disadvantages

- Donor site morbidity from harvest of CFNG
- Potential hemitongue atrophy, speech and mastication deficits, mass activation, and synkinesis with sacrifice of more than 40% of hypoglossal nerve

Masseteric-Facial, Multiple Cross-Face Nerve Grafts

As previously stated, CFNG is the only donor nerve to provide spontaneous, emotive facial function. The timing between reanimation with CFNG and resultant reinnervation is about 6 to 12 months. Thus, in order to use CFNG as the sole nerve transfer, a patient should undergo reanimation as soon as possible in order to reinnervate the facial musculature before muscle atrophy. It is recommended that this occurs within 6 months of injury. If a patient is deemed a candidate for CFNG, multiple CFNGs (zygomatic-zygomatic, buccal-buccal, cervical-marginal) can be performed to restore mimetic function. Typically, the masseteric nerve is coapted to a buccal branch of the nonfunctional facial nerve. If there is no meaningful recovery from the CFNG, hypoglossal-facial nerve transfer can be performed at 1 year postreanimation surgery. Alternatively, one may use the CFNG to power a gracilis flap.

Advantages

- Restoration of spontaneous, mimetic function, and facial tone

Disadvantages

- Donor site morbidity from harvest of CFNG
- Must be performed within 6 months of injury
- CFNG outcomes are not as reliable as masseteric and hypoglossal

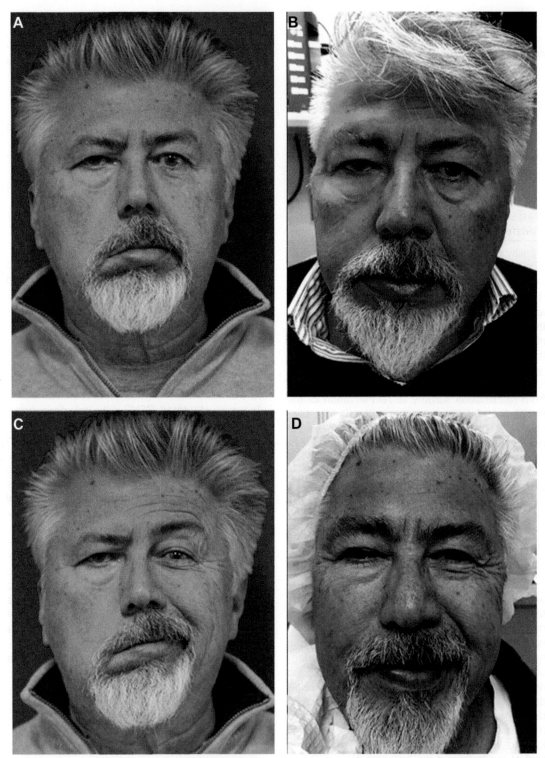

Fig. 6. (*A, B*) Preoperative photos of a patient with right facial nerve paralysis after resection of an acoustic neuroma. Postoperative photos after reinnervation with masseteric, hypoglossal, and CFNG at 11 months (*C*) and 16 months (*D*).

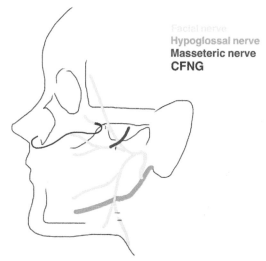

Facial nerve
Hypoglossal nerve
Masseteric nerve
CFNG

Fig. 7. Multiple nerve transfers with the main trunk of the facial nerve are coapted end-to-side to the hypoglossal, the masseteric nerve is coapted to a buccal branch, and a CFNG coapted to a midface branch. Selective cervical branch neurectomy may be performed to reduce synkinesis involving the platysma.

SUMMARY

Nerve substitution is a valuable tool in facial reanimation. Multiple donor nerves have been used for solo and dual innervation. Nerve substitution can also be used as an adjunct to cable grafting to power facial nerve movement. The ideal donor nerve is one that restores dynamic and mimetic facial motion as well was resting facial tone and symmetry.

CLINICS CARE POINTS

- Nerve substitution procedures are indicated when the main trunk of the facial nerve is unavailable for grafting and the distal nerve branches and mimetic muscles are intact.

- Multiple cranial nerves can be used for nerve transfers. It is recommended neurotization surgery be performed within 2 years of injury for best results.

- No donor nerve can guarantee complete facial nerve recovery or restoration of normal facial function.

- Hypoglossal-facial nerve transfer is a popular technique that restores resting facial tone and voluntary smile with neuromuscular training. It is recommended that 40% of the nerve is used in nerve substitution procedures to avoid speech and swallowing deficits, synkinesis, and mass activation.

- Hypoglossal-facial nerve transfer can be performed with an interposition graft from hypoglossal to facial nerve, splitting of 40% of the hypoglossal nerve for end-to-end coaptation, and transposition of the facial nerve from the temporal bone for end-to-side coaptation.

- Masseteric-facial nerve transfer restores voluntary smile, has minimal donor morbidity, does not require an interposition graft, and demonstrates faster recovery when compared with the hypoglossal nerve.

- The major disadvantage of the masseteric nerve is the inability to restore mimetic function and resting facial tone.

- Dual innervation with the masseteric and hypoglossal nerves allows for restoration of resting facial tone from the hypoglossal nerve and creates a more natural smile with clenching, as well as reduced synkinesis from the masseteric nerve.

- The only donor nerve that can restore spontaneous, mimetic function is the contralateral facial nerve. Combining CFNG with dual innervation by the hypoglossal and masseteric nerves allows for recovery of resting facial tone, smile, and mimetic midface and ocular function.

- Masseteric nerve can be used in combination with CFNGs, and cable grafts can allow for faster return of oral commissure movement and minimize synkinesis.

DISCLOSURE

The authors have nothing to disclose.

SUPPLEMENTARY DATA

Supplementary data related to this article can be found online at https://doi.org/10.1016/j.fsc.2021.03.003.

REFERENCES

1. Bascom DA, Schaitkin BM, May M, et al. Facial nerve repair: a retrospective review. Facial Plast Surg 2000;16:309–13.
2. Korte W. Ein Fall von Nervenpfropfung: des Nervus facialis auf den Nervus hypoglossus. Dtsch Med Wochenschr 1903;17:293Y5.
3. Hammerschlag PE. Facial reanimation with jump interpositional graft hypoglossal facial anastomosis and hypoglossal facial anastomosis: evolution in management of facial paralysis. Laryngoscope 1999;109:1–23.

4. May M, Sobol SM, Mester SJ. Hypoglossal-facial nerve interpositional-jump graft for facial reanimation without tongue atrophy. Otolaryngol Head Neck Surg 1991;104:818Y25.

5. Cusimano MD, Sekhar L. Partial hypoglossal to facial nerve anastomosis for reinnervation of the paralyzed face in patients with lower cranial nerve palsies: technical note. Neurosurgery 1994;35(3): 532–3.

6. Slattery WH 3rd, Cassis AM, Wilkinson EP, et al. Side-to-end hypoglossal to facial anastomosis with transposition of the intratemporal facial nerve. Otol Neurotol 2014;35(3):509–13.

7. Spira M. Anastomosis of masseteric nerve to lower division of facial nerve for correction of lower facial paralysis. Plast Reconstr Surg 1978;61:330–4.

8. Brenner E, Schoeller T. Masseteric nerve: a possible donor for facial nerve anastomosis? Clin Anat 1998; 11:396–400.

9. Coombs CJ, Ek EW, Wu T, et al. Masseteric–facial nerve coaptation—an alternative technique for facial nerve reinnervation. J Plast Reconstr Aesthet Surg 2009;62:1580–8.

10. Bianchi B, Ferri A, Ferrari S, et al. The masseteric nerve: a versatile power source in facial animation techniques. Br J Oral Maxillofac Surg 2014;52(3): 264–9.

11. Hontanilla B, Marre D. Comparison of hemihypoglossal nerve versus masseteric nerve transpositions in the rehabilitation of short-term facial paralysis using the Facial Clima evaluating system. Plast Reconstr Surg 2012;130:662e–72e.

12. Yang SF, Xie Y, Kim JC. Outcomes of facial symmetry and tone at rest after masseteric-to-facial nerve transfer. Facial Plast Surg Aesthet Med 2020. [Epub ahead of print].

13. Chen G, Wang W, Wang W, et al. Symmetry restoration at rest after masseter-to-facial nerve transfer: is it as efficient as smile reanimation? Plast Reconstr Surg 2017;140:793–801.

14. Borschel GH, Kawamura DH, Kasukurthi R, et al. The motor nerve to the masseter muscle: an anatomic and histomorphometric study to facilitate its use in facial reanimation. J Plast Reconstr Aesthet Surg 2012;65(3):363–6.

15. Collar RM, Byrne PJ, Boahene KDO. The subzygomatic triangle: rapid, minimally invasive identification of the masseteric nerve for facial reanimation. Plast Reconstr Surg 2013;132:183–8.

16. Owusu JA, Truong L, Kim JC. Facial nerve reconstruction with concurrent masseteric nerve transfer and cable grafting. JAMA Facial Plast Surg 2016; 18:335.

17. Terzis JK, Wang W, Zhao Y. Effect of axonal load on the functional and aesthetic outcomes of the cross-facial nerve graft procedure for facial reanimation. Plast Reconstr Surg 2009;124:1499–512.

18. Dorafshar AH, Borsuk DE, Bojovic B, et al. Surface anatomy of the middle division of the facial nerve: Zuker's point. Plast Reconstr Surg 2013;131(2): 253–7.

Dual Nerve Transfer for Facial Reanimation

Tyler S. Okland, MD[a], Jon-Paul Pepper, MD[b],*

KEYWORDS

- Dual nerve transfer • Facial reanimation • Facial paralysis • Synkinesis • Nerve transfer
- Hypoglossal nerve transfer • Masseteric nerve transfer • Facial nerve

KEY POINTS

- Two commonly used nerve transfer procedures in facial reanimation are facial nerve-to-hypoglossal nerve and masseteric nerve–to–facial nerve transfers.
- Facial nerve-to-hypoglossal nerve transfer yields improvement in resting facial symmetry but minimal excursion of the oral commissure during smile. Masseteric nerve–to–facial nerve transfers improve smile but resting facial symmetry may not be successfully restored.
- Dual nerve transfer efficiently combines transfer of both the masseteric and hypoglossal nerves in a single surgery to improve smile and facial symmetry at rest.

 Video content accompanies this article at http://www.facialplastic.theclinics.com.

INTRODUCTION

Facial paralysis has a negative impact on both appearance and communication[1–3] The surgical options for facial reanimation following facial paralysis are dynamic and evolving, but nerve transfers increasingly are utilized for facial reanimation and generally are recognized as superior to stand-alone cross-facial nerve grafts.[4–6] In this setting, nerve transfer involves coaptation of a regional cranial motor nerve to the nonfunctional facial nerve. The 2 most commonly performed nerve transfers in facial reanimation surgery utilize the hypoglossal and masseteric nerves as regional donors. The hypoglossal nerve–to–facial nerve transfer yields improvement in resting facial symmetry; however, this procedure offers minimal excursion of the oral commissure during smile.[7–9] The masseteric transfer, conversely, provides significant smile restoration but resting facial symmetry may not be restored as successfully in some patients.[10]

In an attempt to restore both oral commissure elevation and improve facial symmetry at rest, the senior author (JPP) recently described a combination of these 2 procedures.[11] The dual nerve transfer for facial paralysis pairs the strengths of regional transfer of both the masseteric and hypoglossal nerves in a single surgery. This article describes the surgical technique and perioperative considerations for this relatively new procedure.

PATIENT SELECTION CRITERIA AND PREOPERATIVE ASSESSMENT

Candidates for the dual nerve transfer procedure have irreversible and complete facial paralysis of a duration of 2 years or less with intact ipsilateral hypoglossal and masseteric donor nerves on clinical examination. If recovery of facial nerve function is uncertain, then electrodiagnostic testing at either 6 months or 12 months after onset of complete paralysis is performed. Given the use of the hypoglossal nerve, patients with clinically

a Department of Otolaryngology–Head and Neck Surgery, Stanford University School of Medicine, Stanford, CA, USA; b Department of Otolaryngology–Head and Neck Surgery, Division of Facial Plastic and Reconstructive Surgery, Stanford Facial Nerve Center, Stanford University School of Medicine, 801 Welch Road, Stanford, CA 94305, USA
* Corresponding author.
E-mail address: jpepper@stanford.edu

Facial Plast Surg Clin N Am 29 (2021) 397–403
https://doi.org/10.1016/j.fsc.2021.03.004
1064-7406/21/© 2021 Elsevier Inc. All rights reserved.

apparent dysphagia or aspiration are not offered treatment via this technique. It should be emphasized clearly that this technique of hypoglossal nerve–to–facial nerve transfer requires complete transection of the nonfunctional facial nerve; therefore, this procedure is reserved for patients who have no prospect for subsequent meaningful recovery of their injured facial nerve without intervention.

In patients with a history of vestibular schwannoma, radiographic assessment of the temporal bone is mandatory. The facial nerve is transected near the second genu. For this reason, surgical access to this region of the nerve must be assured radiographically. Presence of fat grafts that extend into the mastoid or other postsurgical changes from approaches to the lateral skull base must be noted.

Before and after surgery, patients undergo routine clinical assessment that includes the Facial Clinimetric Evaluation (FaCE) questionnaire and Electronic Facial Assessment by Computer Evaluation (eFACE).[12–14] The FaCE questionnaire is a disease-specific patient-reported quality-of-life measure used to assess facial impairment and disability in patients with facial paralysis. It contains 15 statements, each associated with a 5-item Likert scale. Participants select the most appropriate response to prompts, with 1 corresponding to the lowest and 5 to the highest function, used to measure patients' perceptions of specific aspects of their facial impairment and disability. These statements subsequently are grouped into 6 independent domains: social function, facial movement, facial comfort, oral function, eye comfort, and lacrimal control. The overall score is a composite of all domains. Using a specific formula that has been described previously, a score from 0 (worst) to 100 (best) is calculated.[12] The FaCE questionnaire is a validated instrument with excellent internal consistency and test-retest reliability.

The eFACE is a clinician-graded tool that uses 15 visual analog scale scores to evaluate 3 parameters of functional facial function: static symmetry, dynamic movement, and synkinesis. Higher scores in each domain and the total composite score correlate with higher facial function. This assessment tool has been validated as a video-based scoring metric and has high intrarater and interrater reliability. All patients undergoing surgical treatment of facial paralysis are analyzed with these 2 instruments.

SURGICAL TECHNIQUE

Dual nerve transfer is a 2-team surgery in most cases, involving both facial plastic surgery and otologic surgery. Incisions, therefore, include a modified rhytidectomy incision that is extended into both the inframandibular and postauricular creases to provide simultaneous access to the mastoid region, masseteric nerve, and hypoglossal nerve (**Fig. 1**). Blood supply to the auricle is maintained through both an intact superior cutaneous bridge and deep soft tissue connections both preauricularly and via the vascular supply of the ear canal. Coaptation of the second genu of the facial nerve to the hypoglossal nerve is performed first. A mastoidectomy is performed, the facial nerve is decompressed from the fallopian canal, and the nerve is transected near the second genu (**Fig. 2**). The portion of the facial nerve distal to the transection point then is mobilized into the neck. Effective transposition is achieved by dividing the posterior auricular branch of the facial nerve and the fibrous periosteal attachments at the superficial aspect of the stylomastoid foramen. Without these steps, the intratemporal facial nerve may not have sufficient length to reach the hypoglossal nerve.[15,16] In some cases, the posterior belly of the digastric muscle also is divided. The ipsilateral hypoglossal nerve is identified deep to the posterior belly of the digastric muscle. A partial neurotomy is made in the superior aspect of the nerve. The transected facial nerve then is

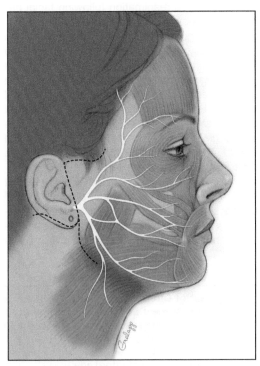

Fig. 1. Illustration of surgical incisions (Illustrations ©Chris Gralapp).

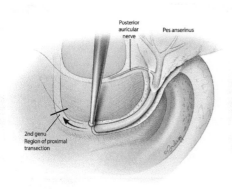

Fig. 2. Location of transection of the facial nerve at the second genu (Illustrations ©Chris Gralapp).

transposed to the hypoglossal nerve and an end-to-side coaptation is completed with 3 interrupted 9-0 nylon sutures, followed by administration of thrombin gel around the coaptation site (**Fig. 3**). All nerve sutures are placed while visualized with an operating microscope.

Through the preauricular incision, the parotid fascia first is identified through a combination of blunt and sharp dissection. This dissection plane then is elevated to the anterior limit of the parotid gland, where the buccal branches of the facial nerve are identified. The desired buccal branch usually is located at a point that is approximately midway between the root of the helix and the ipsilateral oral commissure.[17] Buccal branches in this region are dissected free from the surrounding tissue and preserved as the dissection to the masseteric nerve proceeds. The location of the sigmoid notch is estimated using anatomic measures that previously have been published.[18] At this point, dilute (1:100,000) epinephrine is infused into the sigmoid notch of the mandible, with care not to inject intravascularly. This step aids in characterization of the location of the bony notch that marks

the emergence of the masseteric nerve from the infratemporal fossa and also minimizes bleeding during dissection through the muscle of the masseter. The masseteric nerve is identified near its emergence through the sigmoid notch, coursing anteroinferiorly within the masseter muscle. A nerve stimulator is useful for verification of the nerve because the contraction of the large masseter muscle is robust in response to electrical stimulation of the nerve. It is traced distally to achieve maximum length for transposition and then divided. One of the buccal branches is selected for coaptation, transected proximally, and then coapted to the masseteric nerve using 1 or 2 interrupted 9-0 nylon sutures and thrombin gel (**Fig. 4**). A 10-French round drain is placed prior to incision closure.

CLINICAL OUTCOMES AND DISCUSSION

Two illustrative cases are included. The first is a 42-year-old patient with a history of multiply recurrent right vestibular schwannoma and complete right-sided facial paralysis with a duration of 11 months. Electrodiagnostic testing revealed fibrillation potentials in all muscles tested. She underwent dual nerve transfer, as described previously, and postoperative results 14 months after treatment are shown in **Fig. 5** and Video 1. The patient's FaCE scores improved from 30 to 54 and the composite eFACE score improved from 35 to 71.

The second case is a 55-year-old patient with a history of left-sided vestibular schwannoma with a duration of complete paralysis of 12 months. She previously had undergone upper lid weight placement and limited lateral tarsorrhaphy by an oculoplastic surgeon. After electrodiagnostic testing revealed no evidence of reinnervation, she underwent dual nerve transfer. She underwent dual nerve transfer, as described previously, and postoperative results 25 months after treatment are shown in **Fig. 6** and Video 1. The patient's FaCE scores improved from 33 to 53 and the composite eFACE score improved from 43 to 70.

As discussed previously, the masseteric nerve transfer, when performed in isolation, does not improve resting facial symmetry as effectively as it restores smile. The hypoglossal nerve transfer provides significant improvement in facial symmetry but has a limited capacity to restore a meaningful smile. The authors, therefore, designed a surgical technique to combine the 2 procedures.

Several points are worth noting in the decision-making process with this procedure, because

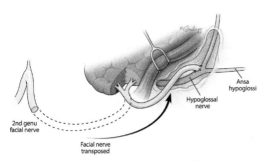

Fig. 3. Facial-to-hypoglossal nerve transfer coaptation (Illustrations ©Chris Gralapp).

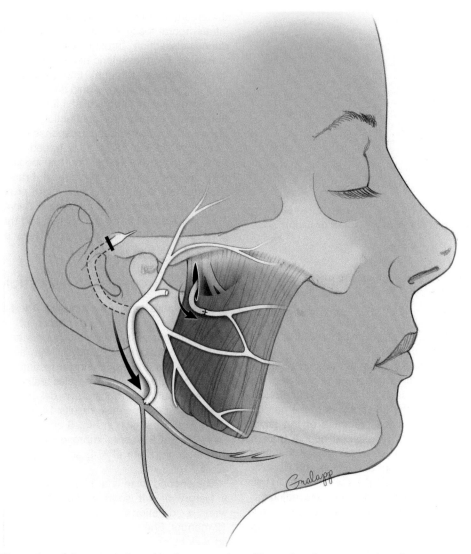

Fig. 4. Illustration of the completion of both masseteric and hypoglossal nerve transfers. The masseteric nerve is coapted end-to-end to a buccal branch of the facial nerve and an end-to-side coaptation of the second genu region of the facial nerve to the hypoglossal nerve. (Illustrations ©Chris Gralapp).

this procedure is but 1 treatment among many surgical treatments for facial paralysis. First, although ipsilateral tongue function is preserved by using a partial neurotomy of the hypoglossal nerve, facial symmetry at rest may not be treated as effectively as restoration of dynamic movement. The degree of contralateral hyperkinesis may vary widely between patients with facial paralysis. Although all patients undergo a course of facial retraining guided by rehabilitation specialists, some patients may have more difficulty matching the movement

of the masseteric nerve transfer to the nonparalyzed side to the reinnervated side of the face. The authors have combined staged cross-facial sural nerve grafting, utilizing the electrical response of the reinnervated facial nerve after dual nerve transfer to map the previously injured nerve and select recipient branches for accurate cross-facial nerve grafting. Lastly, patients with marked contralateral hyperkinesis and dense muscle atrophy alternatively may be treated with fascia lata harvested from the thigh as an

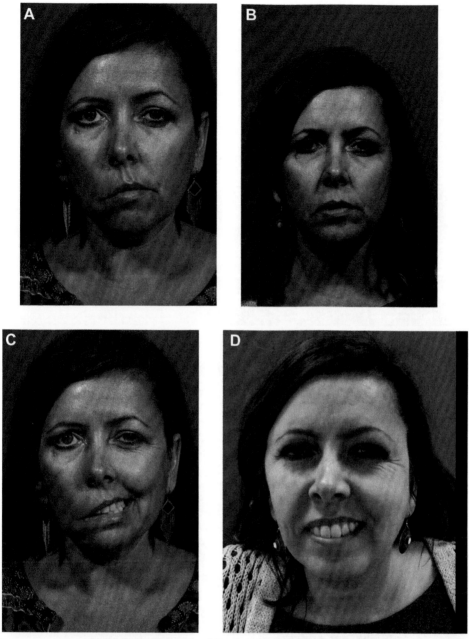

Fig. 5. Pretreatment repose (*A*), smile (*C*) and post-treatment repose (*B*) and smile (*D*) in a 42-year-old patient with a history of multiply recurrent right vestibular schwannoma requiring facial nerve resection for treatment of recurrent tumor. Patient also underwent closed canthopexy and upper lid weight at time of dual nerve transfer surgery.

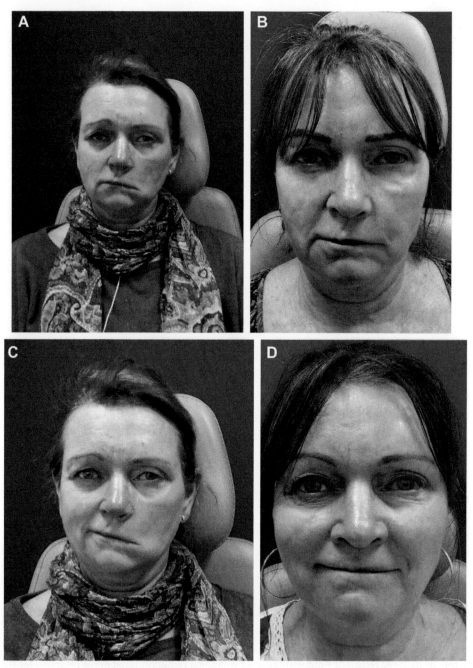

Fig. 6. Pretreatment repose (*A*), smile (*C*) and post-treatment repose (*B*) and smile (*D*) in a 55-year-old patient with a history of multiply recurrent vestibular schwannoma requiring facial nerve transection for treatment of recurrent tumor.

alternative means of reestablishing midfacial symmetry at rest.

CLINICS CARE POINTS

- Patients who are candidates for dual nerve transfer suffer from complete and irreversible facial paralysis and have intact ipsilateral hypoglossal and masseteric nerves without clinical evidence of dysphagia.

- When performing the dual nerve transfer, surgeons must ensure the proximal facial nerve is accessible in cases of prior lateral skull base tumor or surgery.

- Incisions should be planned so as to preserve vascular supply of a superior cutaneous bridge and the deep vascular supply via the external auditory canal.

- A partial, superior neurotomy of the hypoglossal nerve is used to preserve ipsilateral tongue function.

- Patients require postoperative facial retraining in order to maximize their use of the regional nerve transfers.

- Patients with severe contralateral hyperkinesis may require additional or alternative treatments to compensate for the relative strength of the intact facial musculature.

DISCLOSURE

The authors have no conflicts of interest to disclose regarding competing interests, personal financial interests, funding or employment.

REFERENCES

1. Kim JH, Fisher LM, Reder L, et al. Speech and communicative participation in patients with facial paralysis. JAMA Otolaryngol Head Neck Surg 2018;144(8):686–93.
2. Ridgway JM, Crumley RL, Kim JH. Rehabilition of facial paralysis. In: Flint PW, Lund VJ, Haughey BH, et al, editors. Cumming otolaryngology: head and neck surgery. 5th edition. Philadelphia: Elsevier Mosby; 2010. p. 2421–5.
3. Hadlock T. Evaluation and management of the patient with postoperative facial paralysis. Arch otolaryngol Head Neck Surg 2012;138(5):505–8.
4. Klebuc MJ. Facial reanimation using the masseter-to-facial nerve transfer. Plast Reconstr Surg 2011; 127(5):1909–15.
5. Garcia RM, Hadlock TA, Klebuc MJ, et al. Contemporary solutions for the treatment of facial nerve paralysis. Plast Reconstr Surg 2015;135(6):1025e–46e.
6. Mackinnon SE, Novak CB. Nerve transfers. New options for reconstruction following nerve injury. Hand Clin 1999;15(4):643–66, ix.
7. Kochhar A, Albathi M, Sharon JD, et al. Transposition of the Intratemporal facial to hypoglossal nerve for reanimation of the paralyzed face: the VII to XII Transposition technique. JAMA Facial Plast Surg 2016;18(5):370–8.
8. Hontanilla B, Aubá C. Automatic three-dimensional quantitative analysis for evaluation of facial movement. J Plast Reconstr Aesthet Surg 2008;61(1): 18–30.
9. Hontanilla B, Marre D. Comparison of hemihypoglossal nerve versus masseteric nerve transpositions in the rehabilitation of short-term facial paralysis using the Facial Clima evaluating system. Plast Reconstr Surg 2012;130(5):662e–72e.
10. Chen G, Wang W, Wang W, et al. Symmetry restoration at rest after masseter-to-facial nerve transfer: is it as efficient as smile reanimation? Plast Reconstr Surg 2017;140(4):793–801.
11. Pepper JP. Dual nerve transfer for facial reanimation. JAMA Facial Plast Surg 2019;21(3):260–1.
12. Kahn JB, Gliklich RE, Boyev KP, et al. Validation of a patient-graded instrument for facial nerve paralysis: the FaCE Scale. Laryngoscope 2001;111(3):387–98.
13. Banks CA, Bhama PK, Park J, et al. Clinician-graded electronic facial paralysis assessment: the eFACE. Plast Reconstr Surg 2015;136(2):223e–30e.
14. Banks CA, Jowett N, Hadlock TA. Test-retest reliability and agreement between in-person and video assessment of facial mimetic function using the eFACE Facial Grading System. JAMA Facial Plast Surg 2017;19(3):206–11.
15. Campero A, Socolovsky M. Facial reanimation by means of the hypoglossal nerve: anatomic comparison of different techniques. Oper Neurosurg 2007; 61(suppl_3):ONS-41–50.
16. van de Graaf RC, FF IJ, Nicolai JP. Facial reanimation by means of the hypoglossal nerve: anatomic comparison of different techniques. Neurosurgery 2008;63(4):E820.
17. Dorafshar AH, Borsuk DE, Bojovic B, et al. Surface anatomy of the middle division of the facial nerve: Zuker's point. Plast Reconstr Surg 2013;131(2): 253–7.
18. Borschel GH, Kawamura DH, Kasukurthi R, et al. The motor nerve to the masseter muscle: an anatomic and histomorphometric study to facilitate its use in facial reanimation. J Plast Reconstr Aesthet Surg 2012;65(3):363–6.

Facial Reanimation and Reconstruction of the Radical Parotidectomy

Abel P. David, MD, Rahul Seth, MD, Philip Daniel Knott, MD*

KEYWORDS

- Radical parotidectomy • Parotid defects • Facial nerve • Facial reanimation • Reconstruction
- Microvascular surgery

KEY POINTS

- A comprehensive reconstructive approach is required to address the challenges posed by radical parotidectomy, which include rehabilitation of facial paralysis, restoration of facial volume, contour, and symmetry, and attainment of adequate skin coverage.
- Although nerve grafting procedures may provide for optimal facial reanimation, dynamic regional muscle transfer may offer immediate facial symmetry and some expressive movement. Combined approaches of dynamic and static procedures aim to restore immediate facial resting symmetry during or in the absence of reinnervation.
- The anterolateral thigh is a versatile and rich reconstructive donor site that can provide modifiable vascularized soft tissue volume restoration, skin coverage, nerve grafts, and fascia lata grafts for facial reanimation procedures.

INTRODUCTION

Total parotidectomy with facial nerve sacrifice (radical parotidectomy) is performed to treat as many as 20% of parotid gland malignancies when the facial nerve is invaded by a tumor.[1] In addition to facial paralysis, removal of these tumors often leaves patients with significant soft tissue defects of the lateral face and neck and loss of skin coverage. In many cases, postoperative radiation is required to treat these aggressive tumors and should be taken into account when planning the reconstruction. The top priorities for facial reanimation are corneal protection and maintenance of oral competence, followed by restoration of resting symmetry and finally the attainment of dynamic movement. The options for facial reanimation are myriad and include nerve transfer, nerve interposition grafting, static suspension, local muscle transposition, and free tissue transfer. Although reinnervation usually provides the best functional outcomes, its effects may not be noticeable for up to 6 to 12 months.[2,3]

In general, microvascular free flap reconstruction improves blood flow and promotes wound healing in the recipient wound bed, leading to stable soft tissue volumes that are resistant to radiation-induced atrophy.[4] As a part of the oncologic resection, a cervical lymphadenectomy is often performed, providing exposure and access to donor blood vessels for microvascular anastomosis. Additionally, mastoidectomy or lateral temporal bone resection may be necessary because of tumor invasion and/or the need to gain negative surgical margins on proximal perineural tumor spread. It is the authors' preference to approach the reconstruction of the radical parotidectomy defect using a comprehensive approach that starts with the use of the anterolateral thigh (ALT) free flap. This flap offers several key advantages:

Division of Facial Plastic and Reconstructive Surgery, Department of Otolaryngology–Head & Neck Surgery, University of California, San Francisco, 2233 Post Street 3rd Floor, San Francisco, CA 94115, USA
* Corresponding author.
E-mail address: P.Daniel.Knott@ucsf.edu

Facial Plast Surg Clin N Am 29 (2021) 405–414
https://doi.org/10.1016/j.fsc.2021.03.013

Stable and easily modifiable vascularized tissue volume for contour correction,

Vascularized skin for additional cutaneous coverage if needed

Access to tensor fascia lata that can be used for static suspension

Access to the motor nerve to vastus lateralis (MNVL) for cable grafting

Efficiency of a 2-team approach for simultaneous tumor extirpation and flap harvest

Performing an orthodromic temporalis tendon transfer (OTTT) at the time of resection can provide patients with immediate dynamic facial symmetry while awaiting reinnervation. A comprehensive approach also includes performing smaller procedures that address the other consequences of facial paralysis including brow ptosis, lagophthalmos, and ectropion.

FACIAL NERVE RECONSTRUCTION AND REANIMATION

A recent analysis of the National Surgical Quality Improvement Program (NSQIP) database revealed that concurrent facial reanimation and extirpative surgery are performed infrequently, with rates between 24% and 31%.[5,6] It is common practice to defer facial reanimation until after the completion of adjuvant treatment.[6] However, several studies have demonstrated that postoperative radiation and positive nerve margins do not necessarily correlate with adverse nerve reconstruction outcomes.[7–9] Facial reanimation undertaken at the same setting of the extirpation is encouraged, when possible, as facial nerve branches are more easily identified for nerve grafting or nerve transfer, and the duration of facial paralysis and denervation atrophy of facial mimetic muscles are reduced.[6,10]

Nerve Grafting

Depending on the extent of facial nerve resection during a radical parotidectomy, it is usually not feasible to perform a primary coaptation of the proximal and distal nerve segments in a tension-free manner. In these cases, interposition sensory or motor nerve grafts may be used as a method of reinnervation.[11,12] Outcomes do not appear to be significantly affected by adjuvant radiation therapy; patients who underwent nerve grafting and radiation therapy did not have statistically significant outcomes to those who underwent nerve grafting without postoperative radiation.[8,13,14] Some of the more commonly used nerve grafts include the MNVL, cervical sensory nerve, sural nerve, great auricular nerve, lateral antebrachial

cutaneous nerve (LCAN), and the anterior division of the medial antebrachial cutaneous nerve (MACN).[8,13,15] In earlier animal studies, motor nerves grafts appeared to be better suited for motor nerve regeneration compared with sensory nerve grafts. It was hypothesized that this difference is caused by closer matching of the size of the Schwann cell basal lamina tubes, which are larger in motor nerves than in sensory nerves, allowing a greater number of nerve fibers to cross the nerve graft coaptation.[16,17] However, a recent study has refuted this claim and demonstrated equivalent outcomes across 4 validated metrics for motor and sensory nerve grafts in a mouse model.[18] Further research is required to achieve consensus and determine if it also translates clinically. In cases where a suitable nerve graft is not available or to avoid donor site morbidity, cadaveric allografts may be indicated and offer similar outcomes for the reconstruction of sensory, motor, and mixed nerve deficits from 5 to 50 mm.[19]

Functional recovery is optimized when the nerve gap occurs distal to the pes anserinus, with sub-segmental grafting minimizing synkinesis. When the proximal facial nerve is available for nerve grafting, retrograde orientation of the nerve grafts is usually encouraged to minimize axonal escape via regenerating nerves being lost at branch points.[20] However, it is technically difficult to coapt multiple strands to a single facial nerve stump. The MNVL averaged 9.4 cm in length (range 5.1–19.6 cm), and had an average of 4.4 branches, each of which has a mean of 2.3 secondary branches, as shown in a cadaveric study. In vivo, multiple branches (3–5) can often be identified, each of which may be coapted to a distal nerve. This permits efficient single nerve coaptation to the facial nerve trunk, which can then be coapted to multiple distal nerves.[21] For this reason, even when employing the masseteric nerve transfer to the buccal or zygomatic division, the authors encourage the use of the MNVL as an interposition graft during radical parotidectomy. The MNVL is conveniently accessible during an ALT free flap harvest (**Fig. 1**), as the nerve virtually always accompanies the course of the descending branch of the lateral circumflex artery and vein. The MNVL is easily dissected free from the vascular pedicle and has minimal to no associated morbidity because of the apparent redundant innervation of the vastus lateralis.[21] This nerve would be difficult to access for pure nerve grafting procedures in a patient not undergoing an ALT free tissue transfer surgery, as the incision for access would need to be long and the required dissection complicated and time consuming.

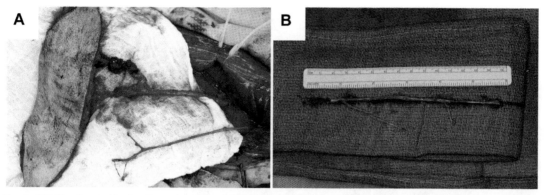

Fig. 1. (A) The donor site for the anterolateral thigh free flap allows access for the simultaneous harvest of the motor nerve to vastus lateralis, (B) nerve to the vastus lateralis with multiple nerve branches.

Nerve to Masseter Transfer

As mentioned previously, in contemporary reconstruction, nerve transfers are increasingly preferred to nerve grafts, because of improved functional recovery associated with higher axonal delivery.[22] Therefore, whether the proximal facial nerve is accessible and given that the distal facial nerve branches are intact and free of tumor, the NTM can be used for subsegmental motor input to either the zygomatic or buccal branches of the facial nerve.[23] The NTM is the largest motor branch of the trigeminal nerve whose number of axon counts match well with the facial nerve.[24] The NTM is reliably found in the subzygomatic triangle, bound by the zygomatic arch (**Fig. 2**), the temporomandibular joint posteriorly, and the frontal branch of the facial nerve.[25] NTM dissection can be started about 3 cm anterior to the tragus and 1 cm to the zygomatic arch, and was found about 1.5 cm deep to the superficial muscular aponeurotic system (SMAS) in this area.[26]

An interesting balancing act is necessary when using combined facial nerve grafts and NTM nerve transfer. Nerve grafts usually offer improved facial tone and limited movement, with some potential synkinesis. The NTM transfer offers greater dynamic commissural excursion, but limited tone. As facial tone is critical for static rest symmetry, and movement is critical for expressivity, an optimal facial reconstructive result would favor the use of both techniques (**Fig. 3**). Other options for facial symmetry at rest include a hypoglossal nerve transfer. Although there were many possible techniques for achieving the hypoglossal-facial nerve transfer (end-to-end or side-to-end), it often calls for transposition of the main trunk of the facial nerve, which is not usually retained during radical parotidectomy. Use of the hypoglossal nerve in radical parotidectomy reconstruction therefore usually requires an interposition nerve graft.[27–29] On the other hand, the NTM is in close proximity to the buccal and zygomatic branches, and a tension-free direct end-to-end coaptation is usually possible, even in extensive facial nerve resections. Engagement of smile excursion is also easier using the NTM, as biting down is a more natural action during smiling than pressing the tongue against the teeth or palate.[30,31] Using the NTM also has minimal morbidity, because the proximal branch of nerve to masseter remains intact, preserving some degree of masseter bulk and function.[23] Uncommonly, patients may experience ocular discomfort while chewing, or masseter atrophy.[31]

Nerve recovery takes about 6 months but can vary depending on patient age and whether the coaptation was to the zygomatic/buccal branch or a facial nerve trunk. Age greater than 40 and facial nerve trunk anastomoses were associated with longer recovery times. Studies of NTM outcomes show patients were afforded an average of 9 mm of oral commissure excursion and as much as 12.5 mm.[31,32]

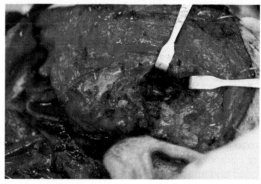

Fig. 2. The nerve to masseter is found within the subzygomatic triangle.

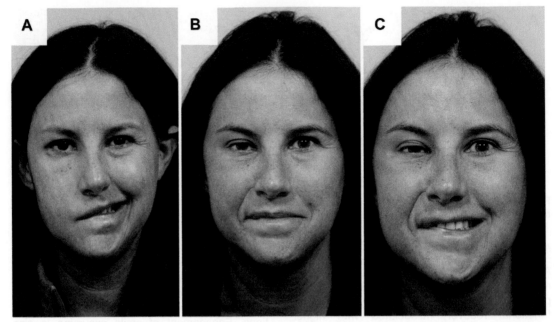

Fig. 3. A patient who underwent a concurrent nerve to masseter transfer and cable grafting demonstrating (*A*) preoperative facial paralysis, (*B*) postoperative resting facial tone, and (*C*) postoperative smile.

Regional Muscle Transfer

The orthodromic temporalis tendon transfer (OTTT) can help immediately restore resting facial symmetry and often commissure excursion and a voluntary, symmetric smile.[33] Performing the temporalis tendon transfer in conjunction with nerve grafting and nerve interposition reduces the duration of loss function while waiting for reinnervation, provides additional movement to reinnervated muscles, and can be used alone when facial nerve recovery is unlikely.[34–36] An OTTT or lengthening temporalis myoplasty (LTM) may easily be performed in conjunction with an ALT flap to permit immediate restoration of tone, movement, and contour.[37]

The temporalis muscle is innervated by the anterior and posterior deep temporal nerves, branches of anterior division of the mandibular nerve (CN V3), and these nerves must be spared during ablative surgery.[38] The temporalis tendon insertion to the coronoid process can be approached via an intraoral or transfacial approach. Often it is accessible through the surgical exposure already provided during a radical parotidectomy. The temporalis tendon is mobilized by first dissecting through the buccal space to expose the coronoid process. Using a sagittal or reciprocating saw, the coronoid may be transected and then transposed and attached near the insertion of the zygomaticus muscles at the corner of the lip. The vector of muscle contraction mimics the zygomaticus

muscle and helps reestablish the melolabial fold.[39] This can immediately restore resting facial symmetry and dynamic reanimation. House and colleagues (2020)[40] reported that patients undergoing OTTT and LTM were able to attain improved static suspension at rest (**Fig. 4**) and nearly 5 mm of oral commissure elevation and 3 mm of horizontal excursion. Patients who would later undergo adjuvant radiation therapy to the parotid bed were able to achieve comparable resting symmetry but had worse commissure excursion and an increased risk of postoperative infection compared with their non-irradiated counterparts.[41] In order to optimize a symmetric and spontaneous smile, patients must undergo postoperative muscle retraining and physical therapy.[42,43]

Static Suspension

For patients with significant comorbidities, absence of a functional trigeminal nerve, or inability to tolerate long durations of general anesthesia, performing dynamic procedures may not be appropriate. Instead, performing static suspension to address oral competence, nasal patency, and nasolabial asymmetry provides immediate results with shorter operative times.[44] Static procedures may be performed to complement nerve grafting and other dynamic procedures. Particular to nerve grafting, static procedures provide functional improvements while awaiting reinnervation.

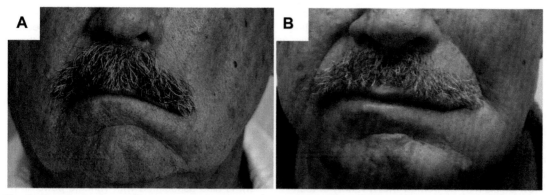

Fig. 4. A patient who underwent a temporalis tendon transfer with a preoperative (*A*) to postoperative (*B*) improvement in resting symmetry, especially of the melolabial fold.

Various grafts and implant materials can be used for these static slings including autologous tissue-like tensor fascia lata,[45] allografts,[44] synthetic grafts,[46] or permanent sutures.[47] Fascia lata grafts are preferred over allografts because of lower rates infection and extrusion.[48] Nonvascularized static suspension grafts should be used with particular caution among patients expected to undergo postoperative radiation therapy, as increased risks of infection are expected. Infected grafts are difficult to salvage, may require removal, and may lead to unsightly scarring or failure of suspension. Static slings are used to suspend the alar base, the nasolabial fold, and the oral commissure to the zygomatic arch or the temporalis fascia (**Fig. 5**).[48] The authors find that it is beneficial to support the lower lip and improve oral competence by suturing fascia lata to the midline lower lip orbicularis muscle and anchoring it to the lateral orbital rim (**Fig. 6**). The immediate cosmetic outcome may suffer because of the need for mild overcorrection but settles as the suspension material gradually stretches over time.[48]

Corneal Protection and Brow Ptosis

The highest priority in the treatment of facial paralysis is corneal protection. Paralysis of the orbicularis oculi muscle results in lagophthalmos and paralytic ectropion, which places the patient at risk for corneal drying and exposure keratitis. Clinicians need to be aware that this potential complication is more likely in the presence of corneal

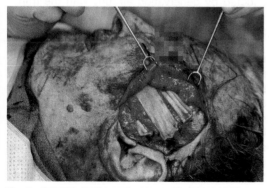

Fig. 5. A patient who underwent a 3-vector static suspension procedure using tensor fascia lata harvested from the lateral thigh.

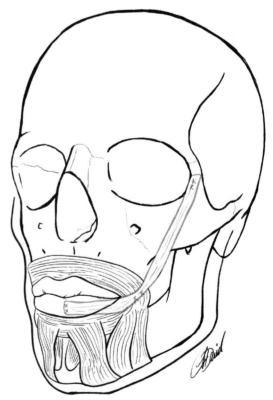

Fig. 6. Depiction of a slip of fascia lata sutured to the midline lower lip orbicularis muscle and anchored to the lateral orbital rim. (*Courtesy of* Abel P. David, MD, San Francisco, CA.)

anesthesia (trigeminal nerve dysfunction), absence of Bell phenomenon, and pre-existing dry eye syndrome. Paralytic lagophthalmos is usually addressed with the placement of an eyelid weight, either made of gold or platinum, and a lower eyelid tightening procedure. Platinum chain eyelid weights are preferred due to lower rates of implant extrusion and lower visibility. They are preferred in cases when long-term paralysis is anticipated.[49–51] Solid (nonchained) weights are more easily removed and may be preferred in patients in whom functional recovery is expected. Brow ptosis may be treated with a variety of techniques, although it is the authors' preference to use trichophytic brow lifts, endoscopic brow lifts, and midforehead brow lifts (**Fig. 7**), depending on the patient's gender, age, hairline, and rhytid patterns such that the paralyzed forehead most closely mirrors the appearance of the contralateral forehead.[52]

VOLUME RESTORATION AND SKIN COVERAGE

Various techniques may be employed to effectively reconstruct the soft tissue volume defects associated with radical parotidectomy. Local flaps, nonvascularized autologous or allograft tissue, and free tissue transfer have all been described. As many options exist, priority must be given to donor site morbidity, reliability, durability, and longevity. Volume deficits with or without temporal bone resection are considerable and have associated aesthetic and social/functional impacts. A study by Anderies and colleagues[53] found that restoration of facial contour following total parotidectomy normalized gaze attentional distraction by tracking eye movements in casual observers.

Locoregional reconstruction options include the sternocleidomastoid flap, the digastric flap, the

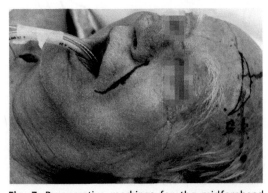

Fig. 7. Preoperative markings for the midforehead brow lift and secondary OTTT.

submental island flap, the supraclavicular artery island flap, the trapezius island flap, and the pectoralis major flap. Local pedicled muscle flaps, besides conferring a variety of donor site morbidities and deformities, also provide short-term muscle bulk that shrinks as the denervated muscle atrophies. Local flaps offer simplicity and oftentimes single-surgeon efficiency, but they must also be raised after the resection is complete, leading to a variable disadvantage in overall operative time.

Nonvascularized parotid bed volume replacement is also associated with variable patterns of success. Acellular dermal allografts and lyophilized dura allografts are associated with considerable ease of use, but confer some associated cost, variable long-term volume stability, and high complication rates.[54,55] Abdominal fat grafting is simple and relatively quick to procure, but is associated with infection, variable long-term stability, and variable ability to withstand external beam radiation. Dermal fat grafts are designed to maximize recipient bed revascularization yet are still associated with infection rates of 8.6% and increasing complications in the setting of external beam radiation.[56]

The anterolateral thigh (ALT) free flap allows for versatility in reconstructing these soft tissue defects, as it can provide sufficient soft tissue volume and skin coverage for even the most extensive radical parotidectomy defects. The vascularized adipofascial flap is favored over local and regional muscle rotational flaps as it is less susceptible to radiation.[57–60] It can be used to refill the volume lost by temporal bone resections, the volume lost by sternocleidomastoid muscle disinsertion, and/or resection and even the volume lost during cervical lymphadenectomy.[61] The soft tissue volume of free muscle flaps, such as gracilis, latissimus dorsi and rectus abdominis, are less reliable and are extensively affected by denervation atrophy with the transferred muscle losing up to 85% to 90% of its post-transfer volume.[62]

In the authors' practice, the ALT free flap is tailored to create contour symmetry to the contralateral side (**Fig. 8**) with a slight overcorrection because of edema caused by the flap harvest. Studies have shown that gross overcorrection is not required because of the stability of the vascularized soft tissue volume, even after exposure to radiation.[63] More recently, Strohl and colleagues (2020) confirmed the stability of adipofascial ALT free flaps even after exposure to radiation therapy. The mean volume after radiation therapy was 96.6% plus or minus 21.7%. Interestingly, they also found that changes in patient body mass

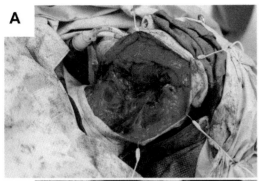

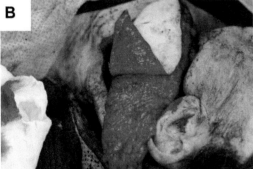

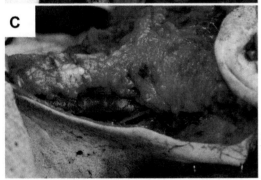

Fig. 8. The anterolateral thigh free flap can be tailored to restore contour defects. In this case, a defect was created by the resection of the sternocleidomastoid muscle (A), the anterolateral thigh free flap be de-epithelialized (B) and shaped to fill the defect (C).

index (BMI) had the greatest association with changes in mean flap volume among all the variables considered.[64]

When feasible and when it does not significantly impede facial reanimation and reestablishing facial symmetry, a buried adipofascial ALT flap can be combined with a cervicofacial advancement flap in order to preserve good color match. Free flaps can be harvested with a skin paddle, which can provide additional skin coverage when extensive skin is resected, but there is color mismatch (**Fig. 9**), especially between the chronic sun-exposed facial skin and the lateral thigh.[65]

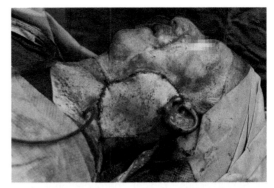

Fig. 9. The skin of the anterolateral thigh free flap is usually lighter than the chronically sun-exposed skin of the face, and therefore there is usually a significant color mismatch.

POSTADJUVANT TREATMENT MANAGEMENT

After the conclusion of adjuvant treatment, facial reanimation procedures can be revised, and the later consequences of continued facial paralysis can be addressed. Eyelid weights can be adjusted/removed; the lower eyelid and brow can be repositioned, and facial contour be refined.[35] After a long period of orbicularis oris paralysis, the lower lip can lengthen, and a wedge excision may be performed to reposition the midline lower lip.[62] In the contralateral face, hyperkinesis can develop and produce involuntary movements exaggerating facial asymmetry. Directed botulinum toxin injections to specific muscles can provide temporary relief.[66–68] Although less noticeable at rest, lower lip paralysis can be emphasized during movement. If patients are satisfied with contralateral botulinum toxin treatment, the normal functioning depressor labii inferioris (DLI) may be sectioned, providing for permanent symmetry.[69] Transposition of the anterior belly of the digastric muscle can be used to reanimate the lower lip depressors. The intermediate tendon of the anterior digastric muscle should be separated from the posterior belly, transposed over the mandible, and sutured to the lateral orbicularis oris muscle.[70]

SUMMARY

Advanced parotid gland malignancies with facial nerve invasion often require aggressive soft tissue resection and facial nerve sacrifice. It is important to consider a patient's comorbidities, the need for adjunctive radiation treatment, and prioritizing certain facial nerve functions when creating a reconstructive plan for the patient. In addition to the rehabilitation of facial paralysis, radical parotidectomy reconstruction must also consider restoring facial contour and symmetry and skin coverage. The authors find that a comprehensive approach that includes the use of the vascularized ALT free flap for stable soft tissue volumes, immediate restoration of resting symmetry and dynamic reanimation with the OTTT, and nerve grafting leads to the most successful functional and aesthetic outcomes.

CLINICS CARE POINTS

- Simultaneous radical parotidectomy and reconstruction occurs infrequently.
- The motor nerve to the vastus lateralis averages 9.4 cm in length and has an average of 4.4 branches.
- Use of the nerve to masseter for facial reanimation leads to an average commissural excursion of 9 mm.
- Use of the temporalis tendon for facial reanimation is associated with 5 mm of commissural elevation and 3 mm of horizontal excursion.
- Use of vascularized adipofascial flaps is associated with atrophy of less than 4% of volume, even after external beam radiation therapy.

DISCLOSURE

The authors have nothing to disclose.

REFERENCES

1. Theriault C, Fitzpatrick PJ. Malignant parotid tumors. Prognostic factors and optimum treatment. Am J Clin Oncol 1986;9(6):510–6.
2. Albathi M, Oyer S, Ishii LE, et al. Early nerve grafting for facial paralysis after cerebellopontine angle tumor resection with preserved facial nerve continuity. JAMA Facial Plast Surg 2016;18(1):54–60.
3. Malik TH, Kelly G, Ahmed A, et al. A comparison of surgical techniques used in dynamic reanimation of the paralyzed face. Otol Neurotol 2005;26(2):284–91.
4. Cannady SB, Seth R, Fritz MA, et al. Total parotidectomy defect reconstruction using the buried free flap. Otolaryngol Head Neck Surg 2010;143(5):637–43.
5. Bovenzi CD, Ciolek P, Crippen M, et al. Reconstructive trends and complications following parotidectomy: incidence and predictors in 11,057 cases. J Otolaryngol Head Neck Surg 2019;48(1):64.
6. Lu GN, Villwock MR, Humphrey CD, et al. Analysis of facial reanimation procedures performed concurrently with total parotidectomy and facial nerve sacrifice. JAMA Facial Plast Surg 2019;21(1):50–5.
7. Hontanilla B, Qiu SS, Marre D. Effect of postoperative brachytherapy and external beam radiotherapy on functional outcomes of immediate facial nerve repair after radical parotidectomy. Head Neck 2014;36(1):113–9.
8. Reddy PG, Arden RL, Mathog RH. Facial nerve rehabilitation after radical parotidectomy. Laryngoscope 1999;109(6):894–9.
9. Wax MK, Kaylie DM. Does a positive neural margin affect outcome in facial nerve grafting? Head Neck 2007;29(6):546–9.
10. Owusu JA, Truong L, Kim JC. Facial nerve reconstruction with concurrent masseteric nerve transfer and cable grafting. JAMA Facial Plast Surg 2016;18(5):335–9.
11. Conley JJ. Facial nerve grafting in treatment of parotid gland tumors; new technique. AMA Arch Surg 1955;70(3):359–66.
12. Millesi H. Nerve grafting. Clin Plast Surg 1984;11(1):105–13.
13. Lee MC, Kim DH, Jeon YR, et al. Functional outcomes of multiple sural nerve grafts for facial nerve defects after tumor-ablative surgery. Arch Plast Surg 2015;42(4):461–8.
14. Pan D, Mackinnon SE, Wood MD. Advances in the repair of segmental nerve injuries and trends in reconstruction. Muscle Nerve 2020;61(6):726–39.
15. Kim J. Neural reanimation advances and new technologies. Facial Plast Surg Clin North Am 2016;24(1):71–84.
16. Nichols CM, Brenner MJ, Fox IK, et al. Effects of motor versus sensory nerve grafts on peripheral nerve regeneration. Exp Neurol 2004;190(2):347–55.
17. Moradzadeh A, Borschel GH, Luciano JP, et al. The impact of motor and sensory nerve architecture on nerve regeneration. Exp Neurol 2008;212(2):370–6.
18. Ali SA, Rosko AJ, Hanks JE, et al. Effect of motor versus sensory nerve autografts on regeneration and functional outcomes of rat facial nerve reconstruction. Sci Rep 2019;9(1):8353.
19. Brooks DN, Weber RV, Chao JD, et al. Processed nerve allografts for peripheral nerve reconstruction: a multicenter study of utilization and outcomes in sensory, mixed, and motor nerve reconstructions. Microsurgery 2012;32(1):1–14.
20. Roberts SE, Thibaudeau S, Burrell JC, et al. To reverse or not to reverse? A systematic review of autograft polarity on functional outcomes following peripheral nerve repair surgery. Microsurgery 2017;37(2):169–74.
21. Revenaugh PC, Knott D, McBride JM, et al. Motor nerve to the vastus lateralis. Arch Facial Plast Surg 2012;14(5):365–8.
22. Murphey AW, Clinkscales WB, Oyer SL. Masseteric nerve transfer for facial nerve paralysis: a systematic review and meta-analysis. JAMA Facial Plast Surg 2018;20(2):104–10.

23. Klebuc M. The evolving role of the masseter-to-facial (V-VII) nerve transfer for rehabilitation of the paralyzed face. Ann Chir Plast Esthet 2015;60(5):436–41.

24. Fournier HD, Denis F, Papon X, et al. An anatomical study of the motor distribution of the mandibular nerve for a masseteric-facial anastomosis to restore facial function. Surg Radiol Anat 1997; 19(4):241–4.

25. Collar RM, Byrne PJ, Boahene KD. The subzygomatic triangle: rapid, minimally invasive identification of the masseteric nerve for facial reanimation. Plast Reconstr Surg 2013;132(1):183–8.

26. Borschel GH, Kawamura DH, Kasukurthi R, et al. The motor nerve to the masseter muscle: an anatomic and histomorphometric study to facilitate its use in facial reanimation. J Plast Reconstr Aesthet Surg 2012;65(3):363–6.

27. Manni JJ, Beurskens CH, van de Velde C, et al. Reanimation of the paralyzed face by indirect hypoglossal-facial nerve anastomosis. Am J Surg 2001;182(3):268–73.

28. Stennert EI. Hypoglossal facial anastomosis: its significance for modern facial surgery. II. Combined approach in extratemporal facial nerve reconstruction. Clin Plast Surg 1979;6(3):471–86.

29. Volk GF, Pantel M, Streppel M, et al. Reconstruction of complex peripheral facial nerve defects by a combined approach using facial nerve interpositional graft and hypoglossal-facial jump nerve suture. Laryngoscope 2011;121(11):2402–5.

30. Coombs CJ, Ek EW, Wu T, et al. Masseteric-facial nerve coaptation–an alternative technique for facial nerve reinnervation. J Plast Reconstr Aesthet Surg 2009;62(12):1580–8.

31. Murphey AW, Clinkscales WB, Oyer SL. Masseteric nerve transfer for facial nerve paralysis. JAMA Facial Plast Surg 2018;20(2):104.

32. Klebuc MJ. Facial reanimation using the masseter-to-facial nerve transfer. Plast Reconstr Surg 2011, 127(5):1909–15.

33. Owusu Boahene KD. Temporalis muscle tendon unit transfer for smile restoration after facial paralysis. Facial Plast Surg Clin North Am 2016;24(1): 37–45.

34. Ciolek PJ, Prendes BL, Fritz MA. Comprehensive approach to reestablishing form and function after radical parotidectomy. Am J Otolaryngol 2018; 39(5):542–7.

35. Fritz M, Rolfes BN. Management of facial paralysis due to extracranial tumors. Facial Plast Surg 2015; 31(2):110–6.

36. Burkhalter WE. Early tendon transfer in upper extremity peripheral nerve injury. Clin Orthop Relat Res 1974;104:68–79.

37. Revenaugh PC, Knott PD, Scharpf J, et al. Simultaneous anterolateral thigh flap and temporalis tendon transfer to optimize facial form and function after radical parotidectomy. Arch Facial Plast Surg 2012; 14(2):104–9.

38. Parker NP, Eisler LS, Dresner HS, et al. Orthodromic temporalis tendon transfer: anatomical considerations. Arch Facial Plast Surg 2012;14(1):39–44.

39. Boahene KD, Farrag TY, Ishii L, et al. Minimally invasive temporalis tendon transposition. Arch Facial Plast Surg 2011;13(1):8–13.

40. House AE, Han M, Strohl MP, et al. Temporalis tendon transfer/lengthening temporalis myoplasty for midfacial static and dynamic reanimation after head and neck oncologic surgery. Facial Plast Surg Aesthet Med 2021;23(1):31–5.

41. Griffin GR, Abuzeid W, Vainshtein J, et al. Outcomes following temporalis tendon transfer in irradiated patients. Arch Facial Plast Surg 2012;14(6):395–402.

42. Coulson SE, Adams RD, O'Dwyer NJ, et al. Physiotherapy rehabilitation of the smile after long-term facial nerve palsy using video self-modeling and implementation intentions. Otolaryngol Head Neck Surg 2006;134(1):48–55.

43. Lambert-Prou MP. [The temporal smile. Speech therapy for facial palsy patients after temporal lengthening myoplasty]. Rev Stomatol Chir Maxillofac 2003;104(5):274–80.

44. Winslow CP, Wang TD, Wax MK. Static reanimation of the paralyzed face with an acellular dermal allograft sling. Arch Facial Plast Surg 2001;3(1):55–7.

45. Rose EH. Autogenous fascia lata grafts: clinical applications in reanimation of the totally or partially paralyzed face. Plast Reconstr Surg 2005;116(1): 20–32 [discussion 33-25].

46. Konior RJ. Facial paralysis reconstruction with Gore-Tex soft-tissue patch. Arch Otolaryngol Head Neck Surg 1992;118(11):1188–94.

47. Alam D. Rehabilitation of long-standing facial nerve paralysis with percutaneous suture-based slings. Arch Facial Plast Surg 2007;9(3):205–9.

48. Langille M, Singh P. Static facial slings: approaches to rehabilitation of the paralyzed face. Facial Plast Surg Clin North Am 2016;24(1):29–35.

49. Becker FF. Lateral tarsal strip procedure for the correction of paralytic ectropion. The Laryngoscope 1982;92(4):382–4.

50. Bianchi B, Ferri A, Leporati M, et al. Upper eyelid platinum chain placement for treating paralytic lagophthalmos. J Craniomaxillofac Surg 2014;42(8): 2045–8.

51. Silver AL, Lindsay RW, Cheney ML, et al. Thin-profile platinum eyelid weighting: a superior option in the paralyzed eye. Plast Reconstr Surg 2009;123(6): 1697–703.

52. Cook TA, Brownrigg PJ, Wang TD, et al. The versatile midforehead browlift. Arch Otolaryngol Head Neck Surg 1989;115(2):163–8.

53. Anderies BJ, Dey JK, Gruszczynski NR, et al. Dermal fat grafting to reconstruct the parotidectomy

defect normalizes facial attention. Laryngoscope 2021;131(1):e124–31.

54. Dulguerov N, Makni A, Dulguerov P. The superficial musculoaponeurotic system flap in the prevention of Frey syndrome: a meta-analysis. Laryngoscope 2016;126(7):1581–4.

55. Govindaraj S, Cohen M, Genden EM, et al. The use of acellular dermis in the prevention of Frey's syndrome. Laryngoscope 2001;111(11 Pt 1): 1993–8.

56. Gruszczynski NR, Anderies BJ, Dey JK, et al. Analysis of abdominal dermal-fat grafting to repair parotidectomy defects: an 18-year cohort study. Laryngoscope 2020;130(9):2144–7.

57. Chandarana S, Fung K, Franklin JH, et al. Effect of autologous platelet adhesives on dermal fat graft resorption following reconstruction of a superficial parotidectomy defect: a double-blinded prospective trial. Head Neck 2009;31(4):521–30.

58. Davis RE, Guida RA, Cook TA. Autologous free dermal fat graft. Reconstruction of facial contour defects. Arch Otolaryngol Head Neck Surg 1995; 121(1):95–100.

59. Gooden EA, Gullane PJ, Irish J, et al. Role of the sternocleidomastoid muscle flap preventing Frey's syndrome and maintaining facial contour following superficial parotidectomy. J Otolaryngol 2001; 30(2):98–101.

60. Sakakibara A, Kusumoto J, Sakakibara S, et al. Long-term effects on volume change in musculocutaneous flaps after head and neck reconstruction. J Reconstr Microsurg 2019;35(4):235–43.

61. Naunheim M, Seth R, Knott PD. Sternocleidomastoid contour restoration: an added benefit of the anterolateral thigh free flap during facial reconstruction. Am J Otolaryngol 2016;37(2):139–43.

62. Ch'ng S, Ashford BG, Gao K, et al. Reconstruction of post-radical parotidectomy defects. Plast Reconstr Surg 2012;129(2):275e–87e.

63. Higgins KM, Erovic BM, Ravi A, et al. Volumetric changes of the anterolateral thigh free flap following adjuvant radiotherapy in total parotidectomy reconstruction. Laryngoscope 2012;122(4):767–72.

64. Strohl MP, Junn JC, House AE, et al. Long-term stability of vascularized adipofascial flaps in facial reconstruction. Facial Plast Surg Aesthet Med 2020;22(4):262–7.

65. Fritz MA, Rolfes BN. Microvascular reconstruction of the parotidectomy defect. Otolaryngol Clin North Am 2016;49(2):447–57.

66. Chen CK, Tang YB. Myectomy and botulinum toxin for paralysis of the marginal mandibular branch of the facial nerve: a series of 76 cases. Plast Reconstr Surg 2007;120(7):1859–64.

67. Conley J, Baker DC, Selfe RW. Paralysis of the mandibular branch of the facial nerve. Plast Reconstr Surg 1982;70(5):569–77.

68. de Maio M, Bento RF. Botulinum toxin in facial palsy: an effective treatment for contralateral hyperkinesis. Plast Reconstr Surg 2007;120(4):917–27 [discussion 928].

69. Lindsay RW, Edwards C, Smitson C, et al. A systematic algorithm for the management of lower lip asymmetry. Am J Otolaryngol 2011;32(1):1–7.

70. Tan ST. Anterior belly of digastric muscle transfer: a useful technique in head and neck surgery. Head Neck 2002;24(10):947–54.

Lessons from Gracilis Free Tissue Transfer for Facial Paralysis: Now versus 10 Years Ago

Matthew Q. Miller, MD*, Tessa A. Hadlock, MD

KEYWORDS

- Facial paralysis • Facial palsy • Gracilis flap • Gracilis free tissue transfer • Smile reanimation

KEY POINTS

- Masseteric-driven free gracilis muscle transfer (FGMT) reliably produces a voluntary smile.
- Cross-face nerve graft (CFNG)-driven FGMT can produce a spontaneous smile, but with a higher risk of failure.
- Dual-innervation FGMT attempts to combine the reliability of masseteric-driven procedures with the spontaneity of CFNG; some element of spontaneity is achieved in approximately 50% of cases.
- Current innovations revolve around re-creating natural smile vectors, improving midface symmetry by performing simultaneous static techniques, avoiding bulk, minimizing scarring, improving spontaneity, and increasing reliability.
- Outcome standardization, pooled data collection, and remote data acquisition methods will be critical to continued improvement of FGMT outcomes.

INTRODUCTION

History

The smile is an evolutionarily adaptive facial expression that facilitates complex social interactions. People smile to convey sympathy, happiness, sociability, and positive intentions toward others.[1,2] Further, people perceive smiling faces as having increased happiness, intelligence, and social standing.[3–6] Hence, smile restoration is a critical component of successful facial reanimation.

Functional muscle transfer has been central to smile restoration since first being described by Sir Harold Gillies.[7] In 1976, Harii and colleagues[8] described using the deep temporal nerve to innervate the first free gracilis muscle transfer (FGMT) for smile reanimation. In 1980, O'Brien and colleagues described cross-face nerve graft (CFNG)-driven FGMT, and since then, the hypoglossal, spinal accessory, and masseteric nerves have been used to innervate transferred gracilis muscle.[9–11]

Most recently, dual-innervation FGMT using the masseteric nerve and a CFNG have been used to produce a spontaneous *and* reliable smile.[10]

A decade ago, FGMT had unclear success rates in producing a smile; limited data demonstrated highly variable outcomes.[12–17] Trigeminally-driven smiles increased in popularity, and ultimately the combination of multiple neural sources emerged as a potential reanimation strategy. This review discusses recent advances in FGMT technique and outcomes reporting.

Key Definitions

FGMT outcomes assessment must consider innervation and vector design. In *masseteric-driven* FGMT, the ipsilateral masseteric branch of cranial nerve V3 is coapted to the anterior branch of the obturator nerve, providing proximal neural input. An anterior branch of the masseteric nerve is preserved, when possible, to prevent

---

The authors have nothing to disclose.
Division of Facial Plastic and Reconstructive Surgery, Department of Otolaryngology, Massachusetts Eye and Ear Infirmary, Harvard Medical School, 243 Charles Street, Boston, MA, USA
* Corresponding author.
E-mail address: matthew_miller@meei.harvard.edu

Facial Plast Surg Clin N Am 29 (2021) 415–422
https://doi.org/10.1016/j.fsc.2021.03.001
1064-7406/21/© 2021 Elsevier Inc. All rights reserved.

asymmetry from muscle atrophy. In *CFNG-driven* FGMT, a healthy-side facial nerve branch that produces a pleasing smile innervates the gracilis, typically via a CFNG placed 6 to 9 months earlier. Direct neurotization without a graft is possible, although outcomes data are limited.[18] *Dual-innervation* FGMT uses the ipsilateral masseteric nerve and a CFNG to power the gracilis. *Dual-vector* (aka multivector) FGMT uses 2 muscle paddles supplied by a common neurovascular pedicle, attempting to recreate natural smile vectors.

HISTORIC OBSTACLES TO SUCCESSFUL SMILE REANIMATION WITH THE GRACILIS FLAP
Unreliability of Cross-Face Nerve Graft–Driven Free Gracilis Muscle Transfer

CFNG-driven FGMT is significantly more likely to produce a spontaneous smile compared with alternative neural sources.[19–24] Unfortunately, these procedures have higher failure rates. O'Brien and colleagues[11] originally reported 51% of patients achieved a smile after CFNG-driven FGMT, and more recent data demonstrate CFNG-driven procedures account for 71% of FGMT failures. Further, CFNG-driven FGMT produces less oral commissure (OC) excursion compared with masseteric-driven procedures.[11,13,25,26]

Lack of Spontaneity in Masseteric-Driven Free Gracilis Muscle Transfer

Masseteric-driven FGMT has excellent reliability; up to 95% of patients produce a smile after surgery.[13,25–27] Despite this excellent reliability, masseteric-driven procedures have low success rates at producing a spontaneous smile.[19,20,24] Historically, lack of spontaneity in masseteric-driven FGMT, along with inconsistent outcomes in CFNG-driven procedures, forced patients and providers to choose between a procedure with high success rates versus a procedure that could produce a spontaneous smile, but with a greater chance of failure.

Cross-Face Nerve Graft–Driven Free Gracilis Muscle Transfer Triggered by Eye Closure

Rarely, CFNG-driven FGMT only produces a smile with eye closure, leading to suboptimal outcomes (**Fig. 1**). This inappropriate smile trigger likely results from incorrect donor nerve selection during first-stage CFNG. Nerve selection can be difficult, as both nerve caliber and muscle movements elicited by nerve stimulation must be considered when selecting healthy-side donor facial nerve branch(es).

Dynamic Success but Poor Aesthetic Outcome

Data typically report changes in OC excursion after FGMT, despite lack of correlation between this measurement and joy conveyed by smiling.[25,26,28] In **Fig. 2**, excellent OC excursion is seen after FGMT, but the smile appears unnatural because of superior malpositioning of the lower lip (**Fig. 2**). Historically, surgeons often focused on maximizing OC excursion rather than re-creating natural smile vectors.

Suboptimal FGMT outcomes can also result from midfacial asymmetry. Midfacial bulk after FGMT can be disfiguring, and patients may avoid smiling to prevent dynamic asymmetry (**Fig. 3**). In 1984, Manktelow and Zuker[29] described transferring a "fascicular territory" of gracilis muscle to decrease bulk. Six years later, in situ muscle thinning was described as another strategy to decrease bulk while minimizing risk for facial hematoma.[30] Despite these techniques, Terzis and Noah[31] reported a 26% revision rate to debulk gracilis muscle in their 1997 case series.

Other factors can also contribute to facial asymmetry after FGMT. Although lymphedema is a widely accepted outcome associated with head and neck cancer therapies, it also likely contributes to midfacial asymmetry in FGMT as large facial and neck flaps are raised.[32] Inappropriate facial contours and hollowing, secondary to fat atrophy and buccal fat prolapse, also can occur after FGMT.

DISCUSSION

Meticulous data collection and outcomes assessment are critical to resolving pitfalls of FGMT. Comprehensive facial paralysis outcomes assessments, which allow comparison among innovations designed to address and resolve these pitfalls, include patient-reported outcome measures, automated analyses, clinician grading, layperson assessments, and spontaneity evaluation.[33]

Addressing Lack of Spontaneity with Masseteric-Driven Free Gracilis Muscle Transfer and High Failure Rate with Cross-Face Nerve Graft–Driven Free Gracilis Muscle Transfer

Ideally, FGMT will combine reliability of masseteric-driven procedures with spontaneity of CFNG-driven FGMT. Dual-innervation FGMT, in which the gracilis is innervated by the masseteric nerve (end-to-end coaptation) and a CFNG (end-to-side coaptation), was described by Biglioli and colleagues[34] to optimize reliability *and* spontaneity. Other neural coaptation patterns since described include Y-shaped and interfascicular

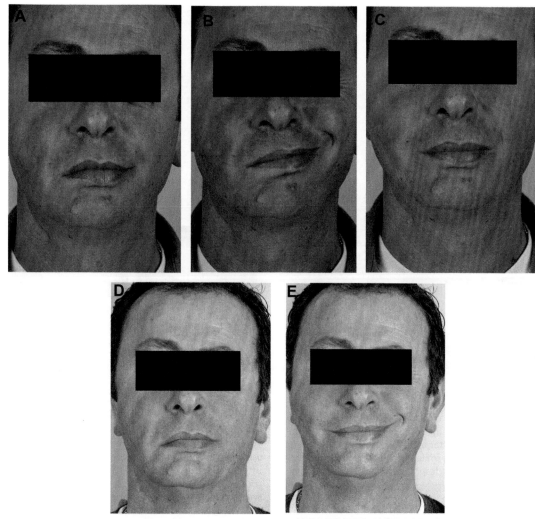

Fig. 1. CFNG-driven FGMT triggered by eye closure. Patient with right facial palsy. *Top row*: 2 years after CFNG-driven FGMT at rest (*left*), attempted smile (*middle*), and tight eye closure (*right*). Note right OC movement with tight eye closure but no movement with attempted smile. *Bottom row*: 16 months after conversion to masseteric-driven FGMT. Patient at rest (*left*) and bite-driven smile (*right*).

split.[24] Rigorous testing of dual-innervation FGMT demonstrates 33% of patients achieve a spontaneous smile, compared with 75% of patients who demonstrate spontaneity after CFNG-driven procedures.[24] A recent review demonstrated higher rates of spontaneity after dual-innervation FGMT, but testing was not standardized.[35] Reliability of dually innervated flaps is excellent.[24,34,36,37] Critical and standardized assessment of dual-innervation FGMT would clarify optimal coaptation pattern(s), and 1-stage versus 2-stage procedure outcomes.[24]

An attractive strategy that may find clinical application in the near future is to provide patients with a reliable and spontaneous smile is a neuroprosthetic device, yoking the paretic hemiface to the healthy side. Implantable neuroprosthetic devices have been developed to treat hearing loss, obstructive sleep apnea, and improve control of prosthetic limbs.[38–42] Multiple groups have demonstrated successful stimulation of paralyzed facial muscles using signals from the healthy hemiface in animal models.[43–48] Devices also must prevent undesirable facial movements during activation to be clinically practical. Jowett and colleagues[49] delivered high-frequency alternating current to the proximal facial nerve to inhibit this undesirable activity, without affecting distal nerve stimulation. Future work should continue to investigate long-term use of implantable neuroprosthetic devices to drive desirable facial movements.

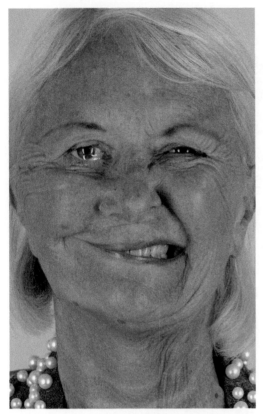

Fig. 2. Excellent OC excursion but superior malpositioning of the lower lip with smile. Patient with right facial palsy 7 years after masseteric-driven FGMT. Note unnatural appearing smile with superior malpositioning of the lower lip, despite excellent OC excursion.

Re-creating a Natural Smile

FGMT has benefited from improved understanding of characteristics that define a natural smile. Boahene and colleagues[50] described multivector FGMT to recreate the zygomaticus *and* levator labii muscles. A multivector approach has also been described for smile reanimation using serratus anterior and sterno-omohyoid free muscle transfers.[51,52] Preliminary work to introduce multivector muscle slips suggests that improved smile morphology may be achieved using this surgical strategy.

Historically, a commonly used FGMT inset technique involved securing the muscle primarily at the modiolus to animate the upper and lower lateral lip. However, this creates unnatural superior malpositioning of the lower lip with smile (see **Fig. 2**). A modified medial inset secures the muscle across the upper lip, from modiolus to philtrum, to improve dental show and create a more natural smile (**Figs. 4 and 5**).[53] Outcomes produced by these new inset and multivector techniques should

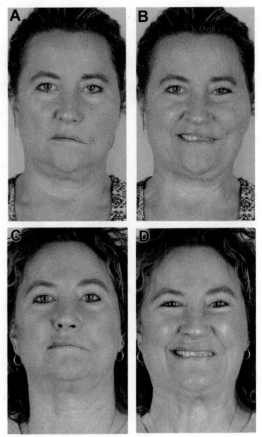

Fig. 3. Midfacial bulk in woman with left facial paralysis after dual-innervation FGMT. *Top row:* 10 months after initial FGMT at rest (*left*) and smile with biting (*right*). Note how asymmetry is more pronounced with smiling. *Bottom row:* 9 months after midfacial debulking and release of gracilis inset from lower lip. Note improved symmetry at rest and with smile after revision procedure.

be evaluated using prior outcomes as control groups.

Preventing and Treating Midfacial Asymmetry

FGMT can introduce midfacial bulk leading to suboptimal aesthetic outcomes. Typical weights of gracilis muscle transplanted 10 to 20 years ago were 25 to 40 g.[54] One recent case series demonstrated 41% of patients with FGMT have excessive midfacial bulk postoperatively. The average flap weight in their series was 33.9 g for CFNG-driven gracilis FGMT and 31.7 g in masseteric-driven flaps.[55] Prior work does not demonstrate a one-to-one correlation between gracilis flap weight and midfacial asymmetry.[26]

The ideal weight of transplanted gracilis muscle remains unknown. Muscle transplants between 25 to 40 g were popular in the 1990s; weights have decreased the past 2 decades to less than 15 g.

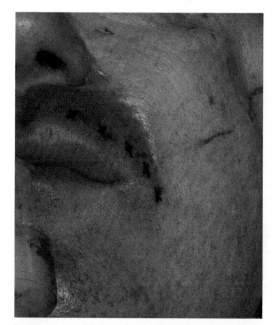

Fig. 4. New medial muscle inset suture locations to improve dental show. Five 0-0 Vicryl sutures are placed in the location of the orbicularis oris from the modiolus to philtrum. No lower lip sutures are placed.

Flaps can be thinned in vivo, as described by O'Brien and colleagues,[30] to minimize hematoma risk. Muscle thinning techniques have been refined so that individual perforators are identified and sealed with surgical clips or bipolar cautery to further minimize hematoma risk.

Although avoidance of bulk and muscle malposition is most desirable, revision procedures can be performed to debulk muscle and/or correct a malpositioned OC when necessary. Muscle thinning in the zygoma region is critical, as bulk is accentuated in this area. Braig and colleagues[55] noted a significant decrease in OC excursion after flap thinning, but improved overall symmetry at rest and

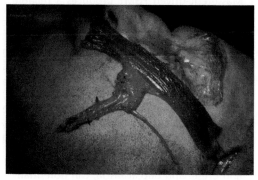

Fig. 5. Muscle laid on face in new medial inset orientation. Note medial edge inset from modiolus to philtrum to improve dental display.

with smile. Greene and colleagues[56] noted improved midfacial symmetry and quality of life in patients who underwent gracilis debulking, without a significant decrease in OC excursion. Repositioning procedures to correct a malpositioned OC also did not affect smile excursion in this series.[56]

Strategies to potentially decrease postoperative lymphedema include shortening the neck incision used for flap inset, and decreasing cautery when raising the facial flap. This shorter incision also minimizes scarring. During facial flap dissection, it is important to preserve the buccal fat pad fascia. If this fascia is violated, it should be reapproximated intraoperatively to prevent postoperative prolapse.

A final strategy to improve *resting* symmetry after FGMT is use of fascia suspension techniques. Our experience has demonstrated that gracilis inset provides adequate OC and lower nasolabial fold (NLF) static suspension in most patients. However, further static correction of the external nasal valve, upper NLF, and philtrum is often needed. A potential strategy to provide this suspension is a single wide band of fascia lata shaped medially to attach to the philtrum, upper NLF, and nasal valve (**Fig. 6**).

Currently, strategies to improve midface symmetry after FGMT largely rely on surgeon experience, because high-quality objective data require long-term follow-up to assess final aesthetic and patient-reported outcomes. As remote follow-up methods improve, optimal size of transplanted muscle and other techniques to prevent midfacial asymmetry should be clarified.

Preventing and Addressing Cross-Face Nerve Graft–Driven FGMT Triggered by Eye Closure

During first-stage CFNG, careful dissection prevents neuropraxia and preserves ability to stimulate facial nerve branches intraoperatively. This intraoperative stimulation is critical to identifying proper donor branch(es) for CFNG. When CFNG-driven FGMT smile is only triggered by eye closure, the CFNG coaptation can be taken down and the obturator nerve reused for coaptation to the masseteric nerve. This sacrifices spontaneity but provides the patient with control of his or her smile.

SUMMARY

Improved data collection methods and critical outcomes assessment have helped advance FGMT technique and results. However, facial reanimation surgeons continue to address pitfalls.

Masseteric-driven FGMT is reliable, but does not produce a spontaneous smile without significant patient adaptation. Dual-innervation FGMT has excellent reliability with varying reported

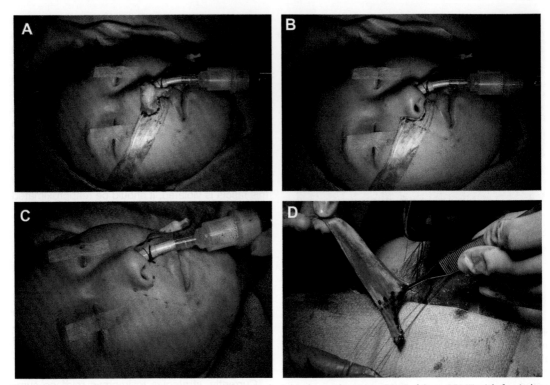

Fig. 6. Fascia lata static suspension. Patient with right facial palsy undergoing CFNG-driven FGMT with fascia lata static suspension. Single wide band (*upper left*) is harvested and then shaped to fit the nasal valve, philtrum, and superior NLF (*upper right*). Small nicks are made with an 11-blade to pass 4-0 Prolene sutures on a straight Keith needle (*lower left*). The fascia is parachuted into place (*lower right*).

success rates at producing a spontaneous smile. These outcomes require continued study using a validated spontaneous smile assessment tool. New medial inset techniques and multivector paddle designs likely improve dental show and produce a more natural smile, although comparison against historical outcomes is needed. Ideally, dynamic lower lip reanimation techniques will be introduced to recreate the depressor labii inferioris' inferolateral pull with smile.

Because of demonstrated success with FGMT, more institutions are performing these procedures, which improves access for patients, but decreases each institution's numbers. It is unclear whether this dilution of numbers will affect outcomes, but it certainly will demand multi-institutional data collection to ensure FGMT outcomes continue to improve. To facilitate multi-institutional data collection, FGMT outcomes should become standardized and remote patient-submitted data collection methods developed. Artificial intelligence automated analyses will also likely play a role in improving FGMT outcomes assessment.

The inability to smile is a devastating complication of facial paralysis. Smile reanimation has significantly advanced the past decade, largely due to improved FGMT techniques and outcomes

assessment tools. Continued surgical advancements, outcome standardization, pooled data collection, and remote outcome assessment tools will help smile reanimation and FGMT continue to progress in the coming decade.

CLINICS CARE POINTS

- Masseteric-driven FGMT produces a reliable *voluntary* smile.

- CFNG-driven FGMT produces a *spontaneous* smile, but has higher failure rates compared with masseteric-driven procedures.

- Preliminary evidence suggests dual-innervation FGMT is reliable and produces a spontaneous smile in approximately 50% of patients.

- Midfacial bulk and asymmetry associated with FGMT can be disfiguring. Lower-weight flaps, shorter neck incisions, and meticulous facial flap dissection, minimizing cautery and preserving buccal fascia, can potentially prevent this asymmetry.

- OC excursion, smile angle, and dental show combine to produce natural, aesthetically pleasing smiles. Multivector gracilis flaps and medial muscle inset across the upper lip can potentially be used to recreate more natural smiles.

- Outcomes standardization, pooled data collection, remote data acquisition, and artificial intelligence assessment will facilitate FGMT comparative effectiveness research.

REFERENCES

1. Keltner D, Bonanno GA. A study of laughter and dissociation: distinct correlates of laughter and smiling during bereavement. J Pers Soc Psychol 1997; 73(4):687–702.
2. Kudoh T, Matsumoto D. Cross-cultural examination of the semantic dimensions of body postures. J Pers Soc Psychol 1985;48(6):1440–6.
3. Otta E, Lira BB, Delevati NM, et al. The effect of smiling and of head tilting on person perception. J Psychol 1994;128(3):323–31.
4. Otta E, Folladore Abrosio F, Hoshino RL. Reading a smiling face: messages conveyed by various forms of smiling. Percept Mot Skills 1996;82(3 Pt 2):1111–21.
5. LaFrance M. Option or obligation to smile: the effects of power and gender on facial expression. In: Philippo FR, Coats EJ, editors. The social context of nonverbal behavior. New York: Cambridge University Press; 1999. p. 45–70.
6. Schmidt KL, Cohn JF. Human facial expressions as adaptations: evolutionary questions in facial expression research. Am J Phys Anthropol 2001;(Suppl 33):3–24.
7. Gillies H. Experiences with fascia lata grafts in the operative treatment of facial paralysis: (Section of Otology and Section of Laryngology). Proc R Soc Med 1934;27(10):1372–82.
8. Harii K, Ohmori K, Torii S. Free gracilis muscle transplantation, with microneurovascular anastomoses for the treatment of facial paralysis. A preliminary report. Plast Reconstr Surg 1976;57(2):133–43.
9. Terzis JK, Noah EM. Dynamic restoration in Möbius and Möbius-like patients. Plast Reconstr Surg 2003;111(1):40–55.
10. Goldberg C, DeLorie R, Zuker RM, et al. The effects of gracilis muscle transplantation on speech in children with Moebius syndrome. J Craniofac Surg 2003;14(5):687–90.
11. O'Brien BM, Franklin JD, Morrison WA. Cross-facial nerve grafts and microneurovascular free muscle transfer for long established facial palsy. Br J Plast Surg 1980;33(2):202–15.
12. Bianchi B, Copelli C, Ferrari S, et al. Facial animation with free-muscle transfer innervated by the masseter motor nerve in unilateral facial paralysis. J Oral Maxillofac Surg 2010;68(7):1524–9.
13. Bae YC, Zuker RM, Manktelow RT, et al. A comparison of commissure excursion following gracilis muscle transplantation for facial paralysis using a cross-face nerve graft versus the motor nerve to the masseter nerve. Plast Reconstr Surg 2006;117(7):2407–13.
14. Zuker RM, Goldberg CS, Manktelow RT. Facial animation in children with Möbius syndrome after segmental gracilis muscle transplant. Plast Reconstr Surg 2000;106(1):1–8 [discussion 9].
15. Bianchi B, Copelli C, Ferrari S, et al. Facial animation in children with Moebius and Moebius-like syndromes. J Pediatr Surg 2009;44(11):2236–42.
16. Ueda K, Harii K, Asato H, et al. Neurovascular free muscle transfer combined with cross-face nerve grafting for the treatment of facial paralysis in children. Plast Reconstr Surg 1998;101(7):1765–73.
17. Gousheh J, Arasteh E. Treatment of facial paralysis: dynamic reanimation of spontaneous facial expression-apropos of 655 patients. Plast Reconstr Surg 2011;128(6):693e–703e.
18. Kumar PA. Cross-face reanimation of the paralysed face, with a single stage microneurovascular gracilis transfer without nerve graft: a preliminary report. Br J Plast Surg 1995;48(2):83–8.
19. Hontanilla B, Cabello A. Spontaneity of smile after facial paralysis rehabilitation when using a non-facial donor nerve. J Craniomaxillofac Surg 2016; 44(9):1305–9.
20. Yoshioka N, Tominaga S. Masseteric nerve transfer for short-term facial paralysis following skull base surgery. J Plast Reconstr Aesthet Surg 2015;68(6):764–70.
21. Sforza C, Tarabbia F, Mapelli A, et al. Facial reanimation with masseteric to facial nerve transfer: a three-dimensional longitudinal quantitative evaluation. J Plast Reconstr Aesthet Surg 2014;67(10):1378–86.
22. Rozen S, Harrison B. Involuntary movement during mastication in patients with long-term facial paralysis reanimated with a partial gracilis free neuromuscular flap innervated by the masseteric nerve. Plast Reconstr Surg 2013;132(1):110e–6e.
23. Faria JC, Scopel GP, Busnardo FF, et al. Nerve sources for facial reanimation with muscle transplant in patients with unilateral facial palsy: clinical analysis of 3 techniques. Ann Plast Surg 2007;59(1):87–91.
24. Dusseldorp JR, van Veen MM, Guarin DL, et al. Spontaneity assessment in dually innervated gracilis smile reanimation surgery. JAMA Facial Plast Surg 2019;21(6):551–7.
25. Hontanilla B, Olivas J, Cabello A, et al. Cross-face nerve grafting versus masseteric-to-facial nerve transposition for reanimation of incomplete facial paralysis: a comparative study using the FACIAL CLIMA evaluating system. Plast Reconstr Surg 2018;142(2):179e–91e.
26. Bhama PK, Weinberg JS, Lindsay RW, et al. Objective outcomes analysis following microvascular gracilis

transfer for facial reanimation: a review of 10 years' experience. JAMA Facial Plast Surg 2014;16(2):85–92.

27. Oh TS, Kim HB, Choi JW, et al. Facial reanimation with masseter nerve-innervated free gracilis muscle transfer in established facial palsy patients. Arch Plast Surg 2019;46(2):122–8.

28. Dusseldorp JR, Guarin DL, van Veen MM, et al. In the eye of the beholder: changes in perceived emotion expression after smile reanimation. Plast Reconstr Surg 2019;144(2):457–71.

29. Manktelow RT, Zuker RM. Muscle transplantation by fascicular territory. Plast Reconstr Surg 1984;73(5): 751–7.

30. O'Brien BM, Pederson WC, Khazanchi RK, et al. Results of management of facial palsy with microvascular free-muscle transfer. Plast Reconstr Surg 1990;86(1):12–22 [discussion 23-4].

31. Terzis JK, Noah ME. Analysis of 100 cases of free-muscle transplantation for facial paralysis. Plast Reconstr Surg 1997;99(7):1905–21.

32. Tyker A, Franco J, Massa ST, et al. Treatment for lymphedema following head and neck cancer therapy: a systematic review. Am J Otolaryngol 2019;40(5):761–9.

33. Dusseldorp JR, van Veen MM, Mohan S, et al. Outcome tracking in facial palsy. Otolaryngol Clin North Am 2018;51(6):1033–50.

34. Biglioli F, Colombo V, Tarrabia F, et al. Double innervation in free-flap surgery for long-standing facial paralysis. J Plast Reconstr Aesthet Surg 2012;65(10):1343–9.

35. Boonipat T, Robertson CE, Meaike JD, et al. Dual innervation of free gracilis muscle for facial reanimation: what we know so far. J Plast Reconstr Aesthet Surg 2020;73(12):2196–209.

36. Cardenas-Mejia A, Covarrubias-Ramirez JV, Bello-Margolis A, et al. Double innervated free functional muscle transfer for facial reanimation. J Plast Surg Hand Surg 2015;49(3):183–8.

37. Kim MJ, Kim HB, Jeong WS, et al. Comparative study of 2 different innervation techniques in facial reanimation: cross-face nerve graft-innervated versus double-innervated free gracilis muscle transfer. Ann Plast Surg 2020;84(2):188–95.

38. Strollo PJ Jr, Soose RJ, Maurer JT, et al. Upper-airway stimulation for obstructive sleep apnea. N Engl J Med 2014;370(2):139–49.

39. Stango A, Yazdandoost KY, Farina D. Wireless radio channel for intramuscular electrode implants in the control of upper limb prostheses. Conf Proc IEEE Eng Med Biol Soc 2015;2015:4085–8.

40. Merrill DR, Lockhart J, Troyk PR, et al. Development of an implantable myoelectric sensor for advanced prosthesis control. Artif Organs 2011;35(3):249–52.

41. Simmons FB. Electrical stimulation of the auditory nerve in man. Arch Otolaryngol 1966;84(1):2–54.

42. Wilson BS, Dorman MF. Cochlear implants: a remarkable past and a brilliant future. Hear Res 2008;242(1–2):3–21.

43. Kurita M, Takushima A, Muraoka Y, et al. Feasibility of bionic reanimation of a paralyzed face: a preliminary study of functional electrical stimulation of a paralyzed facial muscle controlled with the electromyography of the contralateral healthy hemiface. Plast Reconstr Surg 2010;126(2):81e–3e.

44. Frigerio A, Heaton JT, Cavallari P, et al. Electrical stimulation of eye blink in individuals with acute facial palsy: progress toward a bionic blink. Plast Reconstr Surg 2015;136(4):515e–23e.

45. Rothstein J, Berlinger NT. Electronic reanimation of facial paralysis–a feasibility study. Otolaryngol Head Neck Surg 1986;94(1):82–5.

46. Attiah MA, de Vries J, Richardson AG, et al. A rodent model of dynamic facial reanimation using functional electrical stimulation. Front Neurosci 2017;11:193.

47. Tobey DN, Sutton D. Contralaterally elicited electrical stimulation of paralyzed facial muscles. Otolaryngology 1978;86(5). Orl-812-8.

48. Broniatowski M, Ilyes LA, Jacobs G, et al. Dynamic rehabilitation of the paralyzed face–II. Electronic control of the reinnervated facial musculature from the contralateral side in the rabbit. Otolaryngol Head Neck Surg 1989;101(3):309–13.

49. Jowett N, Kearney R, Knox CJ, et al. Toward the Bionic face: a novel neuroprosthetic device paradigm for facial reanimation consisting of neural blockade and functional electrical stimulation. Plast Reconstr Surg 2019;143(1):62e–76e.

50. Boahene KO, Owusu J, Ishii L, et al. The multivector gracilis free functional muscle flap for facial reanimation. JAMA Facial Plast Surg 2018;20(4):300–6.

51. Sakuma H, et al, Tanaka I, Yazawa M. Multivector functioning muscle transfer using superficial sub-slips of the serratus anterior muscle for longstanding facial paralysis. J Plast Reconstr Aesthet Surg 2019; 72(6):964–72.

52. Vincent AG, Bevans SE, Robiitschek JM, et al. Sterno-omohyoid free flap for dual-vector dynamic facial reanimation. Ann Otol Rhinol Laryngol 2020; 129(2):195–200.

53. Jowett N, Hadlock TA. Free gracilis transfer and static facial suspension for midfacial reanimation in long-standing flaccid facial palsy. Otolaryngol Clin North Am 2018;51(6):1129–39.

54. Lindsay RW, Bhama P, Weinberg J, et al. The success of free gracilis muscle transfer to restore smile in patients with nonflaccid facial paralysis. Ann Plast Surg 2014;73(2):177–82.

55. Braig D, Bannasch H, Stark GB, et al. Analysis of the ideal muscle weight of gracilis muscle transplants for facial reanimation surgery with regard to the donor nerve and outcome. J Plast Reconstr Aesthet Surg 2017;70(4):459–68.

56. Greene JJ, Tavares J, Guarin DL, et al. Surgical refinement following free gracilis transfer for smile reanimation. Ann Plast Surg 2018;81(3):329–34.

Strategies to Improve Cross-Face Nerve Grafting in Facial Paralysis

Simeon C. Daeschler, MD[a], Ronald Zuker, MD, FRCSC[b], Gregory H. Borschel, MD[b],*

KEYWORDS

- Facial paralysis • Facial palsy • Facial reanimation • Cross-face nerve graft • Electrical stimulation
- FK506 • Tacrolimus • Supercharge nerve transfer

KEY POINTS

- Facial reanimation aims to improve static and dynamic facial symmetry by improving the resting muscle tone and dynamic muscle excursion in voluntary and spontaneous smiling.
- A challenge that often remains in facial reanimation surgery is combining sufficient muscle excursion and resting tone with spontaneous emotional expression.
- The viability of the target muscle and the neuronal pathway are essential for functional recovery.
- Providing a sufficient number of nerve fibers for muscle reinnervation may improve functional outcomes.
- Combining multiple axon sources for facial reanimation may capitalize the individual advantages of different donor nerves.

INTRODUCTION AND BACKGROUND

Principles of Cross-Face Nerve Grafting

Cross-face nerve grafting describes a surgical nerve transfer technique that uses one or multiple nerve grafts to reroute donor nerve fibers across the median line of the face in order to reanimate contralateral target muscles in unilateral facial palsy. This facial reanimation technique is preferably used when suitable ipsilateral axon sources are unavailable.

If the proximal facial nerve stump on the paralyzed side cannot be used as an axon source, alternative axon sources may be transferred to the dysfunctional facial nerve in order to achieve reinnervation of the facial musculature. Such alternative axon sources can be nearby located cranial nerves including the hypoglossal nerve, the motor nerve to masseter. and even the accessory nerve.[1,2] Alternatively, because of the symmetric innervation pattern of the mimic musculature by the left and right facial nerve, cross-face nerve grafting allows the surgeon to use the contralateral facial nerve as an axon source in unilateral facial palsy. A cross-face nerve graft can be used to reinnervate the facial musculature either as the main axon source or augmentative as a "supercharging" nerve transfer (distal graft end to the side of the recipient facial nerve) for partially recovered facial nerves.[3] Both procedures, however, require viable target muscles to restore motor function. If viable facial musculature is not available for reinnervation, such as following tumor resection, congenital/developmental syndromes, or long denervation times (>18 months), a free functional muscle transfer may be used to provide

[a] Neuroscience and Mental Health Program, Hospital for Sick Children (SickKids), Toronto, Ontario, Canada;
[b] Division of Plastic and Reconstructive Surgery, Hospital for Sick Children (SickKids), University of Toronto, Toronto, Ontario, Canada
* Corresponding author.
E-mail address: gregory.borschel@sickkids.ca

Facial Plast Surg Clin N Am 29 (2021) 423–430
https://doi.org/10.1016/j.fsc.2021.03.009
1064-7406/21/© 2021 Published by Elsevier Inc.

viable musculature into the paralyzed hemiface.[4] A free muscle flap may be powered by ipsilateral axon sources or by a cross-face nerve graft in a 2-stage procedure. During the first stage, one or more "blind-ending" cross-face nerve grafts are tunneled and banked subcutaneously in the paralyzed hemiface, and the proximal graft end is connected to the contralateral facial donor nerve. Then, the donor nerve fibers are allowed to grow through the nerve graft for 6 to 12 months, depending on the chosen graft length, before a free functional muscle transfer is performed in stage II.[1] In the second stage, the banked distal end of the cross-face nerve graft is connected to the motor nerve of the muscle graft or, if a neural pedicle is unavailable, directly sutured to the muscle to induce its reinnervation.

Therapeutic Goals of Cross-Face Nerve Grafting

Loss of facial nerve function affects the patient's daily life in multiple ways.[5,6] The vulnerable ocular surface loses protection due to incomplete eyelid closure as a result of dysfunctional temporal and/or zygomatic facial nerve branches to the orbicularis oculi muscle. In addition, proximal facial nerve lesions located within the temporal bone may affect the parasympathetic facial nerve fiber population that supplies lacrimal and salivary glands as well as the taste receptors in the anterior two-thirds of the tongue. Parasympathetic facial nerve fiber dysfunction thus may result in insufficient lacrimation and salivation, "crocodile tears," gustatory sweating, and impaired taste.[7] However, arguably the most debilitating dysfunction for an affected patient's daily life and their social interactions is the loss of facial expression.[6,8] Facial palsy not only results in impaired dynamic expression but also disables emotional expression, the ability to spontaneously react to emotional stimuli and to formulate clear speech in daily social interactions. There is also a decrease in static muscle tone, resulting in stigmatizing disfigurement. Facial nerve surgery therefore aims to improve static and dynamic facial symmetry by improving both the resting muscle tone and dynamic muscle excursion in voluntary and spontaneous smiling.

Challenges in Cross-Face Nerve Grafting

A challenge in facial reanimation surgery is combining sufficient muscle excursion and resting tone with the ability to spontaneously elicit an emotional facial response. Although ipsilateral non-VII cranial nerve transfers may restore powerful, voluntary muscle contractions, spontaneous and emotional facial expressions are often lacking.[9] A major advantage of cross-face nerve grafting is the possibility of reanimating the paralyzed face via the contralateral facial nucleus, thereby enabling spontaneous and emotional smiling.[9] However, cross-face nerve grafts can fail to provide meaningful levels of contractility and force in target muscles, and thus static and dynamic asymmetries may remain[9,10]; this may in part be explained by the long regeneration distances and smaller donor motor neuron pools provided by cross-face nerve grafts compared with other sources. As a consequence, a reduced number of donor nerve fibers may reach the target muscles after a prolonged period of denervation compared with nerve transfers that use ipsilateral axonal sources.[2]

DISCUSSION—CONTRIBUTING FACTORS TO FUNCTIONAL RECOVERY AND STRATEGIES TO IMPROVE CROSS-FACE NERVE GRAFTING

Sufficient recovery of muscle function following denervation depends on a variety of factors. Key aspects that, at least to some extent, can be influenced by surgical decision-making are the muscles' viability and receptivity to reinnervation, the number of motoneurons that successfully reconnect to the muscle fibers, and the source of motoneurons used for reinnervation.

Key Changes in Denervated Muscle and Nerve and Surgical Strategies to Maintain Their Viability

The viability of denervated musculature, as well as the motor nerves serving those muscles, is heavily time dependent. Although precise time windows are unknown, clinical guidelines and expert consensus presently suggest a maximum denervation time of 12 to 24 months. At this time, the chances for successful restoration of muscle function decline to a level where most surgeons favor alternative reanimation approaches, as reinnervation is more likely to fail; this is because denervated muscle fibers undergo profound cellular changes in response to denervation, including ionic imbalance,[11,12] decreased resting membrane potential,[13] accelerated protein catabolism,[14] permeabilization of the sarcolemma,[15] and activation of the intracellular inflammatome.[16] With increasing denervation time, the contractile apparatus progressively disintegrates[17,18] and the number of intramuscular mitochondria diminishes,[19] with substantial decreases in contractile force.[20] Simultaneously, the intramuscular capillary bed progressively degenerates in response to denervation,[21] contributing to a hypoxic intramuscular environment and fibrotic remodeling of the denervated muscle.[21] As a consequence, chronic denervation of muscle appears histologically as atrophic muscle fibers with a disorganized contractile apparatus, embedded in a dense meshwork of collagenous fibers and adipocytes.[22,23]

Although some aspects of those degenerative changes, such as muscle mass, seem to be partly reversible by long-running external electrical muscle stimulation programs,[22] attempts to reinnervate the long-term denervated muscle are usually less successful, most likely because the intramuscular neural pathways that are left behind the degenerated native nerve fibers become progressively less permissive for regenerating (donor) nerve fibers. The endoneurial tubes inside denervated nerve segments initially serve as guiding structures for regenerating axons[24] and accommodate bands of proliferating, supportive Schwann cells providing a permissive regeneration environment for regrowing axons.[25] In response to prolonged periods of axonal deprivation ("chronic denervation"), the Schwann cells atrophy and the endoneurial tubes are progressively occluded by collagen filaments.[26,27] This adverse intraneural regeneration environment, in combination with the disintegrated contractile apparatus, may explain the low success rate of delayed reanimation approaches.

To ensure target muscle viability, the denervation time should be reduced to a minimum, which generally implies early diagnosis and timely surgical intervention for procedures that aim at reanimating the paralyzed facial musculature. For long-term denervated muscles, repetitive electrical muscle stimulation may be used to externally induce contractions and thereby, at least in part, maintain the contractile apparatus until donor nerve fibers reach the muscle fibers.[22] However, intramuscular and extramuscular neural pathway degeneration may still be present in electrically stimulated muscles, potentially limiting the merit of this procedure for facial palsy. Alternatively, one well-described strategy is to minimize the denervation time of the dysfunctional facial nerve and muscle by combining a cross-face nerve graft with a "babysitting nerve transfer."[1] An ipsilateral motor nerve, such as a portion of the hypoglossal nerve or the motor nerve to masseter, can be coapted end-to-end or end-to-side to the dysfunctional facial nerve to provide reinnervation and maintain a viable musculature. In the same procedure, a cross-face nerve graft is placed to reroute healthy contralateral facial nerve fibers to the dysfunctional facial nerve as a reverse end-to-side nerve transfer (distal graft end to the side of the dysfunctional facial nerve).[1] By combining cross-face nerve grafts with ipsilateral axon

sources, the time of axonal deprivation can be reduced, and patients may benefit from early restoration of muscle function.[28]

Strategies to Increase the Number of Reinnervating Motoneurons

In facial reanimation surgery, the excursion, symmetry, and spontaneity of muscle contractions are key metrics for satisfactory results. The muscle excursion and thereby the dynamic symmetry depend on the number of motoneurons available for muscle reinnervation. If the muscle is reinnervated by a low number of neurons, muscle function partly recovers but force deficits often remain, presumably due to remaining denervated muscle fibers.[29] Accordingly, muscles with moderate functional recovery tend to show a higher number of atrophic muscle fibers,[30] and conversely, a higher number of transferred facial donor nerve fibers is associated with improved muscle function with regard to symmetry and excursion.[31]

Reverse the nerve graft
A simple measure to increase the chance for donor nerve fibers to reach their target is using the nerve graft in a reversed orientation. This ensures that all endoneurial tubes guide the donor nerve fibers to the opposite end of the graft and thereby the target muscle. If instead the graft is used in its physiologic orientation, some endoneurial tubes may lead to former nerve branches. Such branches could have been cut during graft harvest and thus may not be immediately recognizable to the surgeon. Although it is presently unclear whether the concept of reversed graft orientation actually translates into functional improvements[32] and whether those effect sizes would be detectable with currently available diagnostic tools in a reasonably sized clinical sample, we prefer to use grafts in a reversed orientation based on the before-mentioned considerations.

Select suitable donor nerve branches
In addition, in order to increase the number of neurons that eventually reinnervate the target muscle, the surgeon may use a donor nerve branch with a higher axonal load. Depending on the selected branch of the facial nerve and the proximodistal level of transection, the number of transferred donor nerve fibers can vary by a factor of 20, ranging from approximately 150 to 3000 myelinated axons.[31] Following 10 to 14 months of nerve regeneration after stage I, approximately 20% of the transferred donor nerve fibers are detectable as myelinated axons at the distal end of the nerve graft.[30] However, in the absence of a target muscle, a large proportion of axons that regenerated

through the nerve graft seem to remain in a thinly or unmyelinated stage and mature after the nerve fibers are allowed to reinnervate the transferred muscle graft after stage II.[33]

The relevance of rerouting a sufficient number of axons for muscle reanimation becomes evident when comparing the proportion of afferent and efferent axons in peripheral and cranial nerves. Even in nerves often referred to as "pure motor nerves" (eg, accessory or the phrenic nerve) the proportion of efferent (ie, motor) nerve fibers remains less than 30%.[34] Although this highlights the relevance of afferent input for motor control, it also suggests that only the minority of the transferred facial nerve fibers are motor nerve fibers and thus capable of establishing a functional reconnection to the target muscle. Selecting donor nerve branches of appropriate diameter and axonal load may increase the number of provided motor nerve fibers and thus improve recovery of muscle function. Terzis and colleagues proposed approximately 900 myelinated axons as a reasonable cutoff above which they observed a higher rate of sufficient functional recovery after free functional gracilis transfer.[31] Although greater than 90% of the intraparotid zygomatic nerve branches reliably provide more than 900 axons, the proportion of extraparotid zygomatic nerve branches with comparable axon counts rapidly declines in distal direction.[34] Conversely, larger, proximal nerve branches may bundle axons that innervate different targets and thus lose functional specificity. To intraoperatively define the sweet spot that is neither too proximal, thereby losing specificity, nor too distal, thereby losing axonal load, remains challenging and may be subject to considerable uncertainty. Alternatively, surgeons may combine multiple axon sources for facial reanimation.

Combine multiple axon sources
The concept of supercharging aims to combine functional specificity with sufficient axonal load by combining 2 or more axon sources for a single target. Smaller, contralateral facial nerve branches with high functional specificity but insufficient axonal load may be augmented with strong ipsilateral axon sources. The ipsilateral motor nerve to masseter is an anatomically consistent and reliable donor nerve, containing 2700 myelinated nerve fibers on average,[35] short regeneration distances, and thus rapid restoration of function within 3 to 5 months.[2,36] As a result, the motor nerve to masseter is frequently used to restore mimetic muscle function.[36] Physiologically, the masseter is a strong muscle of mastication. Accordingly, facial muscles that have been

reinnervated by a transferred masseter nerve often show strong contractility and correspondingly high oral commissure excursion, close to the maximum excursion of the healthy side, but often with poor resting tone and less emotional spontaneity.[10,37] Similarly, muscle grafts that are powered by the motor nerve to masseter often maintain a larger volume compared with muscles supplied by a cross-face nerve graft, which may indicate a lower proportion of muscle fibers that remain denervated and thus atrophic in nerve to masseter-powered muscles.[38] Thus, combining a cross-face nerve graft with a strong and reliable axon source can increase the number of reinnervating nerve fibers and thus may optimize functional outcomes in facial reanimation surgery.

Although supercharging strategies mainly aim at a quantitative augmentation of smaller donor nerves, the emerging concept of "dual nerve transfers" combines 2 axon sources to capitalize the qualitative advantages of both donor nerves.[39,40] Beyond cross-face nerve grafting, dual nerve transfers have also been proposed for nonfacial axon sources such as the hypoglossal nerve (good muscle resting tone but limited commissure excursion) with the motor nerve to masseter (good muscle excursion but limited resting tone) for facial reanimation.[39] In conclusion, combining multiple axon sources represents a promising chapter in facial reanimation surgery, and future research may inspire even more nuanced surgical concepts to treat facial palsy.

Enhance axonal regeneration
In addition, strategies to enhance the regeneration of the transferred axons may accelerate the reinnervation process and increase the proportion of neurons that reach the target muscle. Brief electrical stimulation (30–60 minutes, 20 Hz) of the transferred donor nerve, proximal to the coaptation site and immediately after or during nerve repair promotes the initial phase of axonal outgrowth and increases the number of nerve fibers that cross the repair site.[41–43] However, the currently available intraoperative techniques require additional operative time to complete the stimulation protocol and the functional benefit of electrical stimulation in cross-face nerve grafting remains to be determined in ongoing studies. Another promising experimental strategy for enhancing nerve regeneration may be the local microdosing of proregenerative drugs directly at the nerve repair site. A recently developed biodegradable drug delivery system for sustained release of Tacrolimus (FK506) was found to accelerate the rate of axonal regeneration in preclinical nerve repair models with minimal off-target drug accumulation in other

organs when compared with systemic drug delivery.[44–46] Future clinical studies will determine the applicability of local drug delivery systems in peripheral nerve repair and facial reanimation.

Protect the pathway

As the endogenous growth support for the regenerating axons decreases in the distal segments of the nerve graft in response to prolonged axonal deprivation, strategies to maintain Schwann cell viability and prevent endoneurial tube occlusion may enhance nerve fiber growth through cross-face nerve grafts. The concept of distal pathway protection resembles the previously mentioned "babysitting" approach for denervated muscle. By connecting the distal end of the cross-face nerve graft to a small sensory nerve branch (eg, a branch of the infraorbital nerve), cellular constituents of the sensory nerve may repopulate the distal graft and maintain a permissive regeneration environment.[47,48] Despite encouraging preclinical evidence[47,49] and although distal pathway protection of cross-face nerve grafts has been shown to be surgically feasible without any detectable donor side deficit,[48] clinical outcome studies are not yet available.

Similarly, aiming at an enhanced growth support for the regenerating axons on their route to the target muscle, some investigators hypothesize that it may be of advantage to increase the length of the neural pedicle of the free muscle flap at stage II of the procedure and shorten the length of the cross-face nerve graft at stage I proportionately,[2] thus providing the regenerating axons with a fresh regeneration environment and decreases the distance needed to traverse within the banked sensory nerve graft. Although compelling in theory, the ideal "nerve graft to pedicle length ratio" for maintaining an optimized growth environment for the regenerating axons and its clinical benefit remains yet to be determined.

Selecting the Appropriate Donor Nerve for Facial Reanimation

Controllability, symmetry, and spontaneity of facial muscle function following reanimation surgery depend on the source of reinnervating neurons. Although the motor nerve to masseter is a reliable axon source, the jaw closing masseter muscle is usually not involved in emotional expression. This lack of integration into emotional neuronal circuits reflects in a low proportion of patients who regain the ability for spontaneous smile and emotional facial expression when the motor nerve to masseter is used for facial reanimation.[9] To regain spontaneity with nonfacial donor nerves, central neuronal circuits need to undergo substantial reorganization.

Individual subsets of a neuron population previously responsible for the motor control of a single muscle now need to be recruited independently and embedded into multiple, new, and functionally distinct neuronal circuits for mimetic motor control. The ability of the central nervous system to fundamentally reorganize its neuronal circuits is highly age dependent and declines rapidly in adults, potentially hampering the functional outcome of the facial reanimation procedure.[50]

Cross-face nerve grafting may reduce the necessary extent of central reorganization because the "rewired" contralateral facial neurons belong to a population that is already integrated into motor control circuits for mimic and emotional facial expression. From a neurophysiological perspective, the cortical motor control of spontaneous facial expression is primarily organized along a horizontal axis. The facial expression of primary emotions, including happiness, interest, surprise, fear, anger, disgust, contempt, and sadness is controlled independently for the upper and lower part of the face,[51] and this allows infants, and to some extent adults, to display a blend of 2 different emotions simultaneously on the upper and lower face. Commonly observed blends of facial expressions in infants are interest and surprise (raised eyebrows with eye opening) on the upper half of the face, coupled with joy, sadness, or anger on the lower face.[52] In contrast, the expression along the vertical facial axis is symmetric, particularly when positive emotions are expressed.[53] Accordingly, it seems to be challenging to display 2 different emotions in the left and right hemiface simultaneously.[54] This lateral symmetry of emotional expression underpins the suitability of contralateral facial nerve fibers for the restoration of a naturally appearing smile and spontaneity in facial reanimation surgery.

To further increase functional specificity, the nerve surgeon can selectively target subsets of neurons with high functional compatibility with their contralateral target muscle by individually mapping the function of facial donor branches via intraoperative nerve stimulation. As such, muscle co-contractions often resemble familiar activation patterns that frequently occur simultaneously in normal facial expression.[53]

Further, the contractile properties of muscle fibers are (re-)defined by the reinnervating neuron population.[55] Fiber type compositions can differ substantially among different muscles, and thus, muscle fiber composition and consequently the contractile properties may change following nerve transfers.[55] Although the clinical relevance of fiber type composition in facial reanimation surgery is incompletely understood, transferring contralateral facial nerve fibers may theoretically result in closer resemblance to the original fiber type composition and contractile properties compared with alternative donor nerves.[30]

SUMMARY

In conclusion, cross-face nerve grafting enables reanimation of the contralateral hemiface in unilateral facial palsy and may recover a spontaneous smile. Various strategies can be adopted to increase the chances for good functional outcomes by maintaining the viability of the neural pathway and target muscle, increasing the number of reinnervating nerve fibers and selecting functionally compatible donor nerve branches. Beyond that, preclinical research has produced a promising group of novel therapies to further enhance nerve regeneration. Future studies will determine their clinical applicability and therapeutic benefit aiming to further improve patient outcomes and push the boundaries in facial reanimation surgery.

CLINICS CARE POINTS

- A key advantage of cross-face nerve grafting is the ability to use the contralateral facial nerve fiber population, which may enable spontaneous and emotional smiling following facial reanimation surgery.[9]

- Supercharging a dysfunctional but partially recovered facial nerve with a cross-face nerve graft can supplement functional gains and thus increase static and dynamic symmetry even years after injury.[56]

- Oral commissure excursion when smiling often remains less than normal levels (approximately 60% of normal excursion) when a cross-face nerve graft is used, but can return to normal levels when the masseteric nerve is used as an additional input to power the muscle.[10]

- Augmenting a cross-face nerve graft with a nonfacial donor nerve may combine spontaneity and sufficient muscle excursion.[57]

- The number of donor nerve fibers available for muscle reinnervation is positively correlated with muscle force and excursion.[29–31]

- Promising strategies to enhance axonal regeneration following nerve surgery are on the horizon.[41,42,44,47,48]

DISCLOSURE

The authors have nothing to disclose.

REFERENCES

1. Terzis JK, Tzafetta K. The "babysitter" procedure: minihypoglossal to facial nerve transfer and cross-facial nerve grafting. Plast Reconstr Surg 2009; 123(3):865–76.
2. Chuang DC, Lu JC, Chang TN, et al. Using the "Sugarcane Chewing" concept as the directionality of motor neurotizer selection for facial paralysis reconstruction: chang gung experiences. Plast Reconstr Surg 2019;144(2):252e–63e.
3. Frey M, Giovanoli P, Michaelidou M. Functional upgrading of partially recovered facial palsy by cross-face nerve grafting with distal end-to-side neurorrhaphy. Plast Reconstr Surg 2006;117(2):597–608.
4. Fattah A, Borschel GH, Manktelow RT, et al. Facial palsy and reconstruction. Plast Reconstr Surg 2012;129(2):340e–52e.
5. Kim JH, Fisher LM, Reder L, et al. Speech and communicative participation in patients with facial paralysis. JAMA Otolaryngol Head Neck Surg 2018;144(8):686–93.
6. Nellis JC, Ishii M, Byrne PJ, et al. Association among facial paralysis, depression, and quality of life in facial plastic surgery patients. JAMA Facial Plast Surg 2017;19(3):190–6.
7. Boerner M, Seiff S. Etiology and management of facial palsy. Curr Opin Ophthalmol 1994;5(5):61–6.
8. Macgregor FC. Facial disfigurement: problems and management of social interaction and implications for mental health. Aesthetic Plast Surg 1990;14(4):249–57.
9. Biglioli F, Colombo V, Tarabbia F, et al. Recovery of emotional smiling function in free-flap facial reanimation. J Oral Maxillofac Surg 2012;70(10):2413–8.
10. Bae YC, Zuker RM, Manktelow RT, et al. A comparison of commissure excursion following gracilis muscle transplantation for facial paralysis using a cross-face nerve graft versus the motor nerve to the masseter nerve. Plast Reconstr Surg 2006;117(7):2407–13.
11. Kotsias BA, Venosa RA. Sodium influx during action potential in innervated and denervated rat skeletal muscles. Muscle Nerve 2001;24(8):1026–33.
12. Picken JR, Kirby AC. Denervated frog skeletal muscle: calcium content and kinetics of exchange. Exp Neurol 1976;53(1):64–70.
13. Ware F Jr, Bennett AL, Mc IA. Membrane resting potential of denervated mammalian skeletal muscle measured in vivo. Am J Physiol 1954;177(1):115–8.
14. Goldspink DF. The effects of denervation on protein turnover of the soleus and extensor digitorum longus muscles of adult mice. Comp Biochem Physiol B 1978;61(1):37–41.
15. Cisterna BA, Vargas AA, Puebla C, et al. Active acetylcholine receptors prevent the atrophy of

skeletal muscles and favor reinnervation. Nat Commun 2020;11(1):1073.

16. Cea LA, Cisterna BA, Puebla C, et al. De novo expression of connexin hemichannels in denervated fast skeletal muscles leads to atrophy. Proc Natl Acad Sci U S A 2013;110(40):16229–34.

17. Lu DX, Huang SK, Carlson BM. Electron microscopic study of long-term denervated rat skeletal muscle. Anatomical Rec 1997;248(3):355–65.

18. Boncompagni S, Kern H, Rossini K, et al. Structural differentiation of skeletal muscle fibers in the absence of innervation in humans. Proc Natl Acad Sci U S A 2007;104(49):19339–44.

19. Gauthier GF, Dunn RA. Ultrastructural and cytochemical features of mammalian skeletal muscle fibres following denervation. J Cell Sci 1973;12(2): 525–47.

20. Squecco R, Carraro U, Kern H, et al. A subpopulation of rat muscle fibers maintains an assessable excitation-contraction coupling mechanism after long-standing denervation despite lost contractility. J Neuropathol Exp Neurol 2009; 68(12):1256–68.

21. Borisov AB, Huang SK, Carlson BM. Remodeling of the vascular bed and progressive loss of capillaries in denervated skeletal muscle. Anatomical Rec 2000;258(3):292–304.

22. Kern H, Boncompagni S, Rossini K, et al. Long-term denervation in humans causes degeneration of both contractile and excitation-contraction coupling apparatus, which is reversible by Functional Electrical Stimulation (FES): a role for myofiber regeneration? J Neuropathol Exp Neurol 2004;63(9):919–31.

23. Carlson BM. The biology of long-term denervated skeletal muscle. Eur J Transl Myol 2014;24(1):3293.

24. Nguyen QT, Sanes JR, Lichtman JW. Pre-existing pathways promote precise projection patterns. Nat Neurosci 2002;5(9):861–7.

25. Fu SY, Gordon T. The cellular and molecular basis of peripheral nerve regeneration. Mol Neurobiol 1997; 14(1–2):67–116.

26. Röyttä M, Salonen V. Long-term endoneurial changes after nerve transection. Acta neuropathologica 1988;76(1):35–45.

27. Vuorinen V, Siironen J, Röyttä M. Axonal regeneration into chronically denervated distal stump. 1. Electron microscope studies. Acta Neuropathol 1995;89(3):209–18.

28. Kim MJ, Kim HB, Jeong WS, et al. Comparative study of 2 different innervation techniques in facial reanimation: cross-face nerve graft-innervated versus double-innervated free gracilis muscle transfer. Ann Plast Surg 2020;84(2):188–95.

29. van der Meulen JH, Urbanchek MG, Cederna PS, et al. Denervated muscle fibers explain the deficit in specific force following reinnervation of the rat

extensor digitorum longus muscle. Plast Reconstr Surg 2003;112(5):1336–46.

30. Frey M, Happak W, Girsch W, et al. Histomorphometric studies in patients with facial palsy treated by functional muscle transplantation: new aspects for the surgical concept. Ann Plast Surg 1991;26(4): 370–9.

31. Terzis JK, Wang W, Zhao Y. Effect of axonal load on the functional and aesthetic outcomes of the cross-facial nerve graft procedure for facial reanimation. Plast Reconstr Surg 2009;124(5):1499–512.

32. Roberts SE, Thibaudeau S, Burrell JC, et al. To reverse or not to reverse? A systematic review of autograft polarity on functional outcomes following peripheral nerve repair surgery. Microsurgery 2017;37(2):169–74.

33. Jacobs JM, Laing JH, Harrison DH. Regeneration through a long nerve graft used in the correction of facial palsy. A qualitative and quantitative study. Brain 1996;119(Pt 1):271–9.

34. Hembd A, Nagarkar PA, Saba S, et al. Facial nerve axonal analysis and anatomical localization in donor nerve: optimizing axonal load for cross-facial nerve grafting in facial reanimation. Plast Reconstr Surg 2017;139(1):177–83.

35. Borschel GH, Kawamura DH, Kasukurthi R, et al. The motor nerve to the masseter muscle: an anatomic and histomorphometric study to facilitate its use in facial reanimation. J Plast Reconstr Aesthet Surg 2012;65(3):363–6.

36. Murphey AW, Clinkscales WB, Oyer SL. Masseteric nerve transfer for facial nerve paralysis: a systematic review and meta-analysis. JAMA Facial Plast Surg 2018;20(2):104–10.

37. Steele JE, Woodcock IR, Murphy AD, et al. Investigation of the activation of the temporalis and masseter muscles in voluntary and spontaneous smile production. J Plast Reconstr Aesthet Surg 2018;71(7):1051–7.

38. Braig D, Bannasch H, Stark GB, et al. Analysis of the ideal muscle weight of gracilis muscle transplants for facial reanimation surgery with regard to the donor nerve and outcome. J Plast Reconstr Aesthet Surg 2017;70(4):459–68.

39. Pepper JP. Dual nerve transfer for facial reanimation. JAMA Facial Plast Surg 2019;21(3):260–1.

40. Boonipat T, Robertson CE, Meaike JD, et al. Dual innervation of free gracilis muscle for facial reanimation: What we know so far. J Plast Reconstr Aesthet Surg 2020.

41. Brushart TM, Hoffman PN, Royall RM, et al. Electrical stimulation promotes motoneuron regeneration without increasing its speed or conditioning the neuron. J Neurosci 2002;22(15):6631–8.

42. Geremia NM, Gordon T, Brushart TM, et al. Electrical stimulation promotes sensory neuron regeneration

and growth-associated gene expression. Exp Neurol 2007;205(2):347–59.

43. Zuo KJ, Gordon T, Chan KM, et al. Electrical stimulation to enhance peripheral nerve regeneration: Update in molecular investigations and clinical translation. Exp Neurol 2020;332:113397.

44. Tajdaran K, Chan K, Shoichet MS, et al. Local delivery of FK506 to injured peripheral nerve enhances axon regeneration after surgical nerve repair in rats. Acta Biomater 2019.

45. Tajdaran K, Chan K, Zhang J, et al. Local FK506 dose-dependent study using a novel three-dimensional organotypic assay. Biotechnol Bioeng 2019;116(2):405–14.

46. Tajdaran K, Shoichet MS, Gordon T, et al. A novel polymeric drug delivery system for localized and sustained release of tacrolimus (FK506). Biotechnol Bioeng 2015;112(9):1948–53.

47. Placheta E, Wood MD, Lafontaine C, et al. Enhancement of facial nerve motoneuron regeneration through cross-face nerve grafts by adding end-to-side sensory axons. Plast Reconstr Surg 2015; 135(2):460–71.

48. Catapano J, Demsey DR, Ho ES, et al. Cross-face nerve grafting with infraorbital nerve pathway protection: anatomic and histomorphometric feasibility study. Plast Reconstr Surg Glob open 2016;4(9): e1037.

49. Gordon T, Hendry M, Lafontaine CA, et al. Nerve cross-bridging to enhance nerve regeneration in a rat model of delayed nerve repair. PLoS One 2015; 10(5):e0127397.

50. Lundborg G, Rosen B. Sensory relearning after nerve repair. Lancet 2001;358(9284):809–10.

51. Ross ED, Gupta SS, Adnan AM, et al. Neurophysiology of spontaneous facial expressions: I. Motor control of the upper and lower face is behaviorally independent in adults. Cortex 2016;76:28–42.

52. Izard CE, Fantauzzo CA, Castle JM, et al. The ontogeny and significance of infants' facial expressions in the first 9 months of life. Dev Psychol 1995;31(6):997–1013.

53. Ekman P, Hager JC, Friesen WV. The symmetry of emotional and deliberate facial actions. Psychophysiology 1981;18(2):101–6.

54. Ross ED, Reddy AL, Nair A, et al. Facial expressions are more easily produced on the upper-lower compared to the right-left hemiface. Percept Mot Skills 2007;104(1):155–65.

55. Bergmeister KD, Aman M, Muceli S, et al. Peripheral nerve transfers change target muscle structure and function. Sci Adv 2019;5(1):eaau2956.

56. Gordon T, de Zepetnek JET. Motor unit and muscle fiber type grouping after peripheral nerve injury in the rat. Exp Neurol 2016;285:24–40.

57. Sforza C, Frigerio A, Mapelli A, et al. Double-powered free gracilis muscle transfer for smile reanimation: a longitudinal optoelectronic study. J Plast Reconstr Aesthet Surg 2015;68(7):930–9.

Dual Innervation of Free Functional Muscle Flaps in Facial Paralysis

Michael J. Klebuc, MD[a,b,]*, Amy S. Xue, MD[a], Andres F. Doval, MD[a]

KEYWORDS

- Dual innervation • Free functional muscle flap • Facial paralysis • Nerve to masseter
- Cross-face nerve graft

KEY POINTS

- Dual innervation can be used to create a marriage of power and spontaneity in free functional muscle flap smile restoration.
- Multiple patterns of dual innervation have been described using cross-face nerve grafts and nerve to masseter with no specific pattern, demonstrating a distinct advantage at this time.
- The presence of ephaptic nerve conduction may help explain the synergy achieved with dual innervation.

INTRODUCTION

Free functional muscle flaps are a highly effective and widely accepted method of smile restoration in cases of developmental and long-standing facial paralysis. The contralateral facial nerve via a cross-face nerve graft (CFNG) and ipsilateral nerve to masseter (NTM) are the most frequently used sources of innervation, with each donor site possessing a series of strengths and weaknesses. The most beneficial property of CFNGs is their ability to produce spontaneous, emotionally mediated muscle activation. Unfortunately, the commissure excursion produced by free muscle flaps innervated by CFNGs may be weaker than the uninjured side. The technique is well suited to children and young adults; however, the ability to achieve smile symmetry declines with age. No strict age cutoff for the technique has been established; however, many surgeons will transition to an ipsilateral nerve donor (CN V, XII, XI) after the third decade of life. In addition, larger muscle flaps are often used to accommodate for the lower axon densities yielded by CFNGs.

In contrast, the masseteric nerve has a dense population of myelinated axons that can reliably produce powerful commissure excursion when used to innervate free muscle flaps. The reconstruction can be achieved in a single surgery, and small, highly tailored muscle flaps can be used as a result of the high axonal load producing minimal cheek bulk. The Achilles heel of the masseter nerve donor site is its limited ability to produce both resting tone and spontaneous facial motion. There is little doubt that a subset of the population possesses communications between CN V and VII as evidenced by electromyographic (EMG) studies.[1,2] Regardless, the number of individuals that can achieve a truly spontaneous smile with a muscle flap innervated solely by the masseter nerve is limited. Clenching of the teeth is initially required for smile activation; however, with diligent practice over a 2-year period, most patients will not have to bite to elicit motion. In 1 study, 53% of patients thought they could produce a smile without conscious effort, which was accredited to the process of cerebral adaptation.[3] In the authors' experience, the development of an

[a] Institute for Reconstructive Surgery, Houston Methodist Hospital, 6560 Fannin Street, Suite #2200, Houston, TX 77030, USA; [b] Weill Cornell School of Medicine, 1300 York Avenue, New York, NY 10065, USA
* Corresponding author. Institute for Reconstructive Surgery, Houston Methodist Hospital, 6560 Fannin Street, Suite #2200, Houston, TX 77030.
E-mail address: mklebuc@msn.com

Facial Plast Surg Clin N Am 29 (2021) 431–438
https://doi.org/10.1016/j.fsc.2021.03.006

effortless, reflexive smile is common; however, true spontaneous motion arising from the masseteric nerve is rare.

The central question to be answered is whether dual innervation of a free muscle flap with a CFNG and the ipsilateral masseter nerve will produce a functional synergy, creating a marriage of power (CN V) and spontaneity (CN VII).

DISCUSSION

A series of different groups have explored this concept and have taken significantly different approaches in their effort to answer this question. Watanabe and colleagues[4] are widely credited for first reporting dual innervation of free muscle flaps for facial reanimation. Their initial technique used a single-stage free latissimus dorsi flap with coaptation of the thoracodorsal nerve to the contralateral facial nerve. The masseter muscle was denuded and placed in direct contact with the latissimus dorsi muscle to encourage muscle-to-muscle neurotization. The technique has subsequently been modified to include a composite latissimus dorsi-serratus anterior muscle flap to create a dual vector.[4] The thoracodorsal nerve is again anastomosed to a contralateral

facial nerve branch. However, in this technique, a motor nerve branch to masseter is buried into the latissimus dorsi muscle to achieve direct intramuscular neurotization. The long thoracic nerve innervating the associated slip of the serratus anterior is coapted to a second "thin" motor branch to masseter, creating direct nerve-to-nerve neurotization (**Fig. 1**). Small masseter branches and direct muscle neurotization are selected to disadvantage the masseter nerve and prevent it from overwhelming innervation arising from the contralateral facial nerve. Regardless of the style of nerve coaptation, using the masseter nerve in this fashion has the potential to limit muscle atrophy with the one-stage technique, where one must wait for axonal growth through a cross-face nerve segment. Innervation strategies like this could potentially permit the utilization of smaller muscle flaps that create less bulk, which has been a drawback of the one-stage latissimus flap technique.

Biglioli and colleagues[5] have also investigated the potential value of dual innervation. Their technique uses a single-stage free gracilis muscle flap innervated by the masseter and contralateral facial nerve. The obturator nerve is anastomosed end to end to the masseter nerve, and the distal

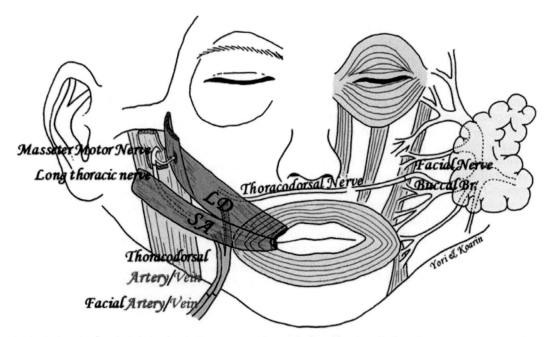

Fig. 1. Composite free latissimus dorsi-serratus anterior muscle flap. The thoracodorsal nerve is anastomosed to a contralateral facial nerve branch. A masseter nerve branch is implanted into the latissimus dorsi muscle, providing intramuscular neurotization. A second masseter nerve branch is coapted to the long thoracic nerve end to end. LD, latissimus dorsi; SA, serratus anterior. (*From* Watanabe Y, Akizuki T, Ozawa T, et al. Dual innervation method using one-stage reconstruction with free latissimus dorsi muscle transfer for re-animation of established facial paralysis: simultaneous reinnervation of the ipsilateral masseter motor nerve and the contralateral facial nerve to improve the quality of smile and emotional facial expressions. J Plast Reconstr Aesthet Surg. 2009;62:1589-1597.)

CFNG is coapted to the obturator nerve end to side (**Fig. 2**). Innervating in this fashion clearly provides a distinct advantage to the masseter nerve with its larger axon load, close proximity, and more efficient anastomosis (end to end). There is a potential concern with this pattern of connections that the masseter nerve will win the race to the motor endplates, crowding out the late-arriving axons from the CFNG. Regardless, this method of dual innervation is most frequently cited in the literature, and this study reports 2 excellent and 2 good results according to the Terzis classification with EMG evidence of gracilis muscle activity with stimulation of the contralateral facial nerve.[6–8] The investigators postulate that the strength of spontaneous muscle contraction may represent axons from the CFNG costimulating the motor nerve fibers from masseter in conjunction with the flaps limited denervation time. The idea of a weaker population of nerve fibers triggering a more robust population is very intriguing and will be explored later in this article.

Cardenas-Mejia and associates[9] have also described using these sources of innervation but in a distinctly different way. A dually innervated free gracilis muscle flap is performed in 2 stages. A CFNG with a proximal end-to-end anastomosis is performed during the first stage. Following successful nerve growth through the graft, the second stage is performed. Here, the CFNG is anastomosed end to end to the obturator nerve, and the masseter nerve is coapted to the obturator nerve end to side approximately 1 cm from the hilum (**Fig. 3**). This configuration is used to optimize the opportunity of the axons from the CFNGs to occupy the flaps motor end plates before arrival of nerve fibers for the masseter nerve. The authors report 9 cases, with Terzis grade 3 achieved in 1 cases, grade 4 achieved in 4 cases, and grade 5 achieved in 4 cases.

Another variation is described by Uehara and Shimizu,[10] who anastomose the masseter nerve end to end to an intramuscular nerve branch in the gracilis while coapting the obturator nerve directly to a CFNG (**Fig. 4**). Dusseldorp and colleagues[11] have also described a two-stage approach where the CFNG and NTM are both anastomosed end to end with the obturator nerve sometimes using an interfascicular split.

The authors' experience with dual innervation began in 2003. The technique was initially used in cases when frozen section evaluation of the previously placed CFNG demonstrated a limited population of axons. In an effort to enhance axonal

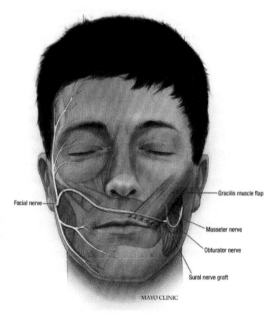

Fig. 2. Single-stage dual innervation of free gracilis muscle flap with the masseter nerve anastomosed to the obturator nerve (end to end) and a CFNG coapted to the obturator nerve (end to side). (*From* Boonipat T, Robertson CE, Meaike JD, et al. Dual innervation of free gracilis muscle for facial reanimation: What we know so far. *J Plast Reconstr Aesthet Surg.* (In press) https://doi.org/10.1016/j.bjps.2020.05.084)

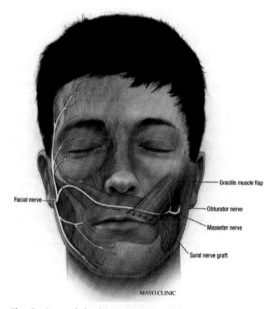

Fig. 3. Staged dual innervation of free gracilis muscle flap with the masseter nerve anastomosed to the obturator nerve (end to side) and the CFNG coapted to the obturator nerve (end to end). (*From* Boonipat T, Robertson CE, Meaike JD, et al. Dual innervation of free gracilis muscle for facial reanimation: What we know so far. *J Plast Reconstr Aesthet Surg.* (In press) https://doi.org/10.1016/j.bjps.2020.05.084)

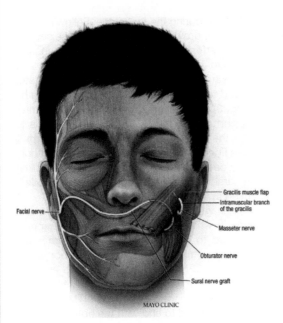

Fig. 4. Dual innervation of free gracilis muscle flap with end-to-end coaptation of CFNG to obturator and end-to-end repair of masseter nerve to intramuscular motor branch. (*From* Boonipat T, Robertson CE, Meaike JD, et al. Dual innervation of free gracilis muscle for facial reanimation: What we know so far. *J Plast Reconstr Aesthet Surg*. (In press) https://doi.org/10.1016/j.bjps.2020.05.084)

input to the free muscle flap, an end-to-end neurorrhaphy was created between the CFNG, NTM, and obturator nerve in a Y configuration. The initial results were somewhat disappointing, as several patients demonstrated improved resting tone. However, a spontaneous smile was not realized, and the commissure excursion was less than what would be anticipated by a flap powered by the NTM alone. It appeared that in the race to the motor end plates the axons arising from the CFNG came in a very distant second. Subsequently, the technique was modified in an effort to disadvantage the masseter nerve. A long segment of obturator nerve is included in the flap design. The fascicular architecture of the transected obturator nerve is mapped. An incomplete neurotomy is made in the obturator nerve near the hilum transecting the dominant fascicles while preserving the integrity of the smaller adjacent fascicles. The CFNG is coapted end to end to the partially divided obturator nerve. The descending branch of the masseter nerve is sutured to the completely transected, proximal obturator nerve end to end, aligning the dominant fascicle in the masseter nerve to the smaller fascicles in the obturator nerve that have not been divided downstream (**Fig. 5**). This connection pattern is used

to maximize axonal load coming from the CFNG while allowing NTM to secondarily populate any unoccupied motor end plates. This two-stage innervation strategy is now offered frequently to older patients seeking free functional muscle smile restoration and is no longer considered a lifeboat option (**Figs. 6** and **7**). In this patient population, end-to-side nerve repairs are also created between infraorbital nerve sensory branches in the lip and the CFNG to enhance Schwann cell viability and maximize axonal growth through the graft.[12]

As demonstrated above, there are multiple dual innervation strategies that differ with regard to staging, muscle flap selection, and nerve coaptation patterns. With such variability in the approach, can an optimal method of dual innervation be identified?

Dusseldorp and associates[11] evaluated 25 patients that had undergone a dually innervated free gracilis muscle flap using 3 different forms of neurorrhaphy (**Fig. 8**). In group 1, the NTM and the CFNG were anastomosed end to end to the obturator nerve after separation of its distal end into 2 fascicular clusters (interfascicular split). In group 2, they were coapted directly to the end of the obturator nerve without interfascicular dissection (Y-shaped neurorrhaphy). The final group underwent a proximal end-to-end repair of the NTM to the obturator and an end-to-side repair of the CFNG to the obturator nerve near the hilum after creating an epineural window. No significant difference was identified in eFACE scores or postoperative commissure excursion between the 3 types of neurorrhaphies. An extensive review of the literature was performed by the Mayo Clinic group, and a total of 57 cases could be identified using many of the dual innervation strategies described above.[6] Terzis scores were recorded in 26 patients who largely demonstrated good to excellent results, and no significant difference was seen whether the NTM was coapted to the obturator nerve end to end and the CFNG end to side or vice versa. They concluded that dual innervation appears safe with muscle flap contraction similar to flaps innervated by the NTM alone. However, the limited number of cases and variable means of reporting make outcome differentiation impractical at this time.

An alternate form of nerve conduction referred to as ephaptic coupling may help explain the lack of variability between the various patterns of dual innervation. With ephaptic conduction, firing of a primary nerve can induce firing of an adjacent nerve, creating secondary excitation. Electrical coupling of adjacent nerve fibers may be caused by ion exchange between cells.[13] Alternately, coupling of nerve fibers may result from the

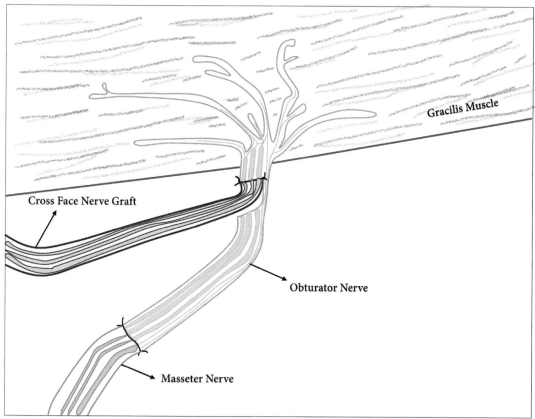

Fig. 5. Staged dual innervation of a free gracilis muscle flap. CFNG coapted end to end to the obturator nerve after creation of a distal neurotomy. Masseter nerve repaired end to end to proximal, long obturator nerve segment.

presence of local electrical fields. Neurons may be ephaptically coupled to local field potentials, creating synchronized conduction.[14] This type of neural excitation has been demonstrated in cases of hemifacial spasm and also helps explain activation of cardia muscle.[15,16] One can imagine a wave of electrical excitation derived from a CFNG washing across a free muscle flap and coactivating the motor units innervated by the NTM. Ephaptic conduction may explain the triggering effect of the CFNG in cases of dual innervation that have been described by several investigators.[4,5,9]

The question remains whether dual innervation can truly produce spontaneity, and if so, how does it compare to flaps innervated solely by

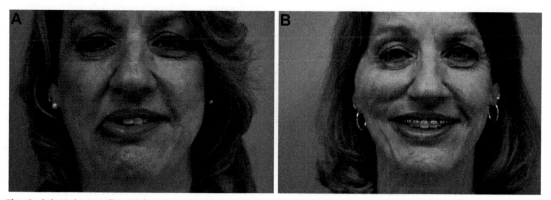

Fig. 6. (*A*) Right nonflaccid facial paralysis and synkinesis after Bell palsy. (*B*) One year after facial reanimation with dual innervated free gracilis muscle flap and right depressor anguli oris myectomy.

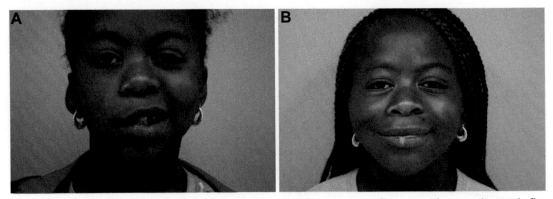

Fig. 7. (*A*) Right developmental facial paralysis. (*B*) Fifth postoperative year after staged free gracilis muscle flap facial reanimation with dual innervation.

CFNGs? This question was investigated in the Mayo Clinic literature review.[6] A total of 36 dual innervated flaps were identified where spontaneity was measured. Of that group, 88% were able to achieve a spontaneous smile similar to muscles innervated by CFNG alone. Unfortunately, there is little uniformity in how spontaneity is evaluated, making these data pieces harder to interpret. Sforza and colleagues[17] analyzed 13 cases of single-stage dual innervation with humorous video and optoelectronic motion tracking technology. Using this technique, they were able to demonstrate spontaneity in 70% of patients. In addition, Kim and associates[18] reported on 31 patients who had received dual innervated gracilis muscle

flaps (1 stage, NTM end to end/CFNG end to side). FACEgram software was used to evaluate smile excursion, symmetry index, and spontaneity. Terzis scoring was also used. A total of 25.8% of the dual innervated group demonstrated spontaneity; however, no significant difference in Terzis scores was noted between dual innervated flaps and those powered by a CFNG alone. A focused evaluation of the ability of dual innervation to produce a spontaneous smile was conducted at the Massachusetts Eye and Ear Infirmary.[11] A novel video time-stamped analysis was used to gauge spontaneous, synchronous commissure movements in response to humorous videos. Some degree of spontaneous smiling was identified in 89%

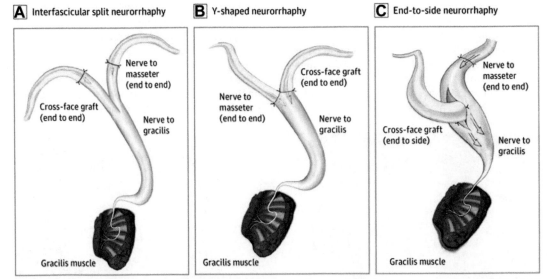

Fig. 8. The patterns of nerve coaptation. (*A*) Masseter and CFNG to obturator end to end after interfascicular split. (*B*) Masseter and CFNG to obturator nerve end to end (Y pattern). (*C*) Masseter to obturator end to end and CFNG to masseter end to side. (*From* Dusseldorp JR, Van Veen MM, Guarin DL, et al. Spontaneity assessment in dually innervated gracilis smile reanimation surgery. *JAMA Facial Plast Surg* (Published on line) October 31, 2019.)

of dual innervate free functional muscle flaps (FFMF). The median percentage of synchronous oral commissure movement as compared with the unaffected side was 33% in the dual innervated group. This percentage drops to 16.5% when one looks exclusively at cases of flaccid facial paralysis with no retained facial motion. This compares with 20% median percentage of synchronous oral commissure movement witnessed in flaps innervated solely by NTM and 75% in those powered exclusively by CFNGs. They concluded that dual innervation performed at least as well as NTM alone. However, isolated CFNGs remained the most reliable technique for creating spontaneity with the proviso that they may produce less commissure excursion than NTM alone and have a higher failure rate.

SUMMARY

In conclusion, there does appear to be value in dual innervating FFMFs especially in the older patient population and when the need to enhance axonal input is encountered. The optimal muscle flap, number of surgical stages, and exact pattern of nerve coaptation have yet to be determined. The role of ephaptic nerve conduction in dual innervated flaps also warrants investigation. The final conclusions regarding dual innervation of FFMFs will likely not be realized until a multi-institutional study with standardized data collection and analysis is performed.

CLINICS CARE POINTS

- Consider dual innervation if frozen section biopsy of cross face nerve graft (CFNG) demonstrates a limited population of axons.
- Consider dual innervation in the older patient population.
- The Nerve to Masseter (NTM) can be identified 3 cm in front of the tragus and 1 cm below the zygomatic arch resting on the deep lobe of the muscle.
- Utilize the descending branch of the NTM to avoid visible muscle atrophy.
- When NTM is the dominant source of innervation a smaller muscle flap can be utilized.

DISCLOSURE

The authors have no financial interest to declare in relation to the content of this article.

REFERENCES

1. Lenz Y, Kiefer J, Dietrich F, et al. Pre-operative masseter muscle EMG activation during smile predicts synchronicity of smile development in facial palsy patients undergoing reanimation with the masseter nerve: a prospective cohort study. J Plast Reconstr Aesthet Surg 2019;72(3):505–12.
2. Schaverien M, Morgan G, Stewart K, et al. Activation of the masseter muscle during normal smile production and the implications for dynamic reanimation surgery for facial paralysis. J Plast Reconstr Aesthet Surg 2011;64:1585–8.
3. Manktelow RT, Tomat LR, Zuker RM, et al. Smile reconstruction in adults with free muscle transfer innervated by the masseter motor nerve: effectiveness and cerebral adaptation. Plast Reconstr Surg 2006;118(4):885–99.
4. Watanabe Y, Akizuki T, Ozawa T, et al. Dual innervation method using one-stage reconstruction with free latissimus dorsi muscle transfer for re-animation of established facial paralysis: simultaneous reinnervation of the ipsilateral masseter motor nerve and the contralateral facial nerve to improve the quality of smile and emotional facial expressions. J Plast Reconstr Aesthet Surg 2009;62:1589–97.
5. Biglioli F, Colombo V, Tarabbia F, et al. Double innervation in free-flap surgery for long-standing facial paralysis. J Plast Reconstr Aesthet Surg 2012;65: 1343–9.
6. Boonipat T, Robertson CE, Meaike JD, et al. Dual innervation of free gracilis muscle for facial reanimation: what we know so far. J Plast Reconstr Aesthet Surg 2020;73(12):2196–209.
7. Boahene KO, Owusu J, Ishii L, et al. The multivector gracilis free muscle functional flap for facial reanimation. JAMA Facial Plast Surg 2018;20(4):300–6.
8. Bianchi B, Ferri A, Copelli C, et al. The masseteric nerve: a versatile power source in facial animation techniques. Br J Oral Maxillofac Surg 2014;52(3):264–9.
9. Cardenas-Mejia A, Covarrubias- Ramirez JV, Bello-Margolis A, et al. Double innervated free functional muscle transfer for facial reanimation. J Plast Surg Hand Surg 2015;49(3):183–8.
10. Uehara M, Shimizu F. The distal stump of the intramuscular motor branch of the obturator nerve is useful for the reconstruction of long-standing facial paralysis using a double-powered free gracilis muscle flap transfer. J Craniofac Surg 2018;29(2):476–81.
11. Dusseldorp JR, Van Veen MM, Guarin DL, et al. Spontaneity assessment in dually innervated gracilis smile reanimation surgery. JAMA Facial Plast Surg 2019;21(6):551–7.
12. Plancheta E, Wood MD, Lafontaine C, et al. Enhancement of facial nerve motoneuron regeneration through cross-face nerve grafts by adding end-to-side sensory axons. Plast Reconstr Surg 2015;135(2):460–71.
13. Ramón F, Moore JW. Ephaptic transmission in squid giant axons. Am J Physiol 1978;234(5):162–9.

14. Stacey RG, Hilbert L, Quail T. Computational study of synchrony in fields and microclusters of ephaptically coupled neurons. J Neurophysiol 2015;113(9):3229–41.

15. Roth BJ. Does ephaptic coupling contribute to propagation in cardiac tissue? Biophys J 2014;106(4): 774–5.

16. Nielsen VK. Electrophysiology of the facial nerve in hemifacial spasm: ectopic/ephaptic excitation. Muscle Nerve 1985;8(7):545–55.

17. Sforza C, Frigerio A, Mapelli A, et al. Double-powered free gracilis muscle transfer for smile reanimation: a longitudinal optoelectronic study. J Plast Reconstr Aesthet Surg 2015;68(7):930–9.

18. Kim MJ, Kim HB, Jeong WS, et al. Comparative study of 2 different innervation techniques in facial reanimation: cross face nerve graft verses double-innervated free gracilis muscle transfer. Ann Plast Surg 2020;84(2):188–95.

Treating Nasal Valve Collapse in Facial Paralysis
What I Do Differently

Jason D. Pou, MD[a],*, Krishna G. Patel, MD, PhD[b], Samuel L. Oyer, MD[c]

KEYWORDS

- Facial paralysis • Nasal obstruction • Nasal valve collapse

KEY POINTS

- Nasal obstruction is a common symptom associated with facial paralysis yet often is overlooked.
- The fundamental discrepancy causing nasal obstruction in patients with flaccid paralysis versus nonflaccid paralysis is inferomedial displacement of the alar base.
- Nasal valve suspension produces superolateral displacement of the ala and is necessary for correcting nasal obstruction in flaccid paralysis.
- The authors' nasal valve suspension technique uses marginal and temporal incisions with fascia lata to produce reliable results without external facial scars.

INTRODUCTION

Patients with facial paralysis require a systematic zonal assessment to assure no areas are overlooked.[1] Flaccid paralysis results from denervation of muscles of facial expression and leads to facial asymmetry from loss of tone and increased skin laxity. One frequently overlooked region is the effect of facial paralysis on nasal airflow.[2] It is important to distinguish flaccid and nonflaccid facial paralysis when assessing nasal obstruction. Patients with nonflaccid paralysis, such as incomplete paralysis with or without synkinesis, typically respond well to cartilage-grafting techniques performed in rhinoplasty. Patients with flaccid paralysis experience increased weight of the cheek as well as loss of muscle tone in the ala and sidewall; this significantly contributes to nasal valve narrowing and collapse.[2–4] These specific findings are often not adequately corrected with traditional functional rhinoplasty-grafting techniques. Successfully treating nasal obstruction in the setting of facial paralysis begins with a thorough history and physical examination. Flaccid paralysis typically results in inferomedial displacement of the alar base, which must be restored with suspension techniques to fully treat the nasal obstruction. Multiple surgical options exist and are discussed in this article.

ANATOMY

The term *nasal valve* was first introduced by Mink in 1903 and was further described in detail by Bridger and Proctor in 1970.[5,6] The internal nasal valve comprises the caudal edge of the upper lateral cartilage, the septum, the head of the inferior turbinate, and the soft tissue overlying the piriform aperture. The internal nasal valve angle is created by the caudal edge of the upper lateral cartilage and the septum; this angle should measure 10° to 15° but varies with ethnicity. The internal nasal valve is the narrowest portion of the nasal cavity and contributes at least 50% of nasal airflow resistance. The external nasal valve is the area delineated by the nostril rim. Medially, it is defined by the medial crus of the lower lateral cartilage and

[a] Facial Plastic and Reconstructive Surgery, Department of Otolaryngology, Head and Neck Surgery, Ochsner Medical Center, 2820 Napoleon Avenue, Suite 820, New Orleans, LA 70115, USA; [b] Facial Plastic and Reconstructive Surgery, Department of Otolaryngology, Head and Neck Surgery, Medical University of South Carolina, 135 Rutledge Avenue, MSC 550, Charleston, SC 29425, USA; [c] Facial Plastic and Reconstructive Surgery, Department of Otolaryngology, Head and Neck Surgery, University of Virginia, PO Box 800713, Charlottesville, VA 22908, USA
* Corresponding author.
E-mail address: Jasonpou4@gmail.com

Facial Plast Surg Clin N Am 29 (2021) 439–445
https://doi.org/10.1016/j.fsc.2021.03.012

columella. Inferiorly, it is bound by the nasal sill and floor of the nose. Laterally, the external valve consists of the alar sidewall.

The alar sidewall is commonly referred to as the "fibrofatty tissue of the ala"; this is the most compliant portion of the nose because of lack of cartilage support. However, there is significant muscle activity that supports and stents the nasal ala and sidewall.[3] The dilator naris muscle occupies a large majority of the ala and plays an important role in opening and strengthening the external valve. The alar portion of the nasalis muscle (pars alaris) inserts on accessory cartilage and influences lateral stability of the ala. The transverse portion of the nasalis (pars transversalis) does not directly insert onto the nasal cartilage but stabilizes the nasal valve and sidewall while acting on the nasal skin[3,7] (**Fig. 1**).

An additional important structure within the alar subunit is the piriform ligament. The piriform ligament is a fibrous ligamentous attachment that extends from the lateral crura to the piriform crest. This structure provides further stability to the alar sidewall; however, it may act as a limiting factor when surgically widening the alar base. This retaining ligament can be divided for complete mobilization.[8]

PHYSIOLOGY

The nose acts as a dynamic airflow resistor. As inspired air enters the nose, the airflow travels superiorly, and its speed increases 5-fold within the internal nasal valve. This region makes up for 50% or more of the total airway resistance. The airflow becomes turbulent, enhancing warming and humidification. Posterior to the nasal valve, the airflow decreases to approximately its entrance speed and turns horizontally and then inferiorly toward the choanae. The airflow becomes laminar and increases speed as it enters the nasopharynx.[8]

Nasal airflow follows the principle explained by Bernoulli. A liquid or gas flowing through a tube increases its velocity and diminishes the transmural pressure at an area of constriction. The Bernoulli effect explains why the nasal valve collapses at varying degrees of nasal inspiration. Three factors determine the amount of nasal valve collapse with inspiration: the shape of the nasal valve area, the cross-sectional area of the nasal valve, and the integrity of the nasal sidewall and ala.[8] Poiseuille's law states that flow is inversely related to the radius to the fourth power, which explains why a slight decrease is nasal valve area results in a dramatic decrease in nasal airflow.

EVALUATION OF NASAL OBSTRUCTION

When evaluating patients with facial paralysis, a systematic approach should be implemented. When focusing on nasal obstruction, a thorough history focusing on the nasal symptoms will help one determine the fundamental problem. Understanding the effect of nasal obstruction on the patient's quality of life is important to determine the appropriate management option. Patient-based quality-of-life surveys focusing on facial palsy (Facial Clinimetric Evaluation Scale, Facial Disability Index) and on nasal obstruction (Nasal Obstruction and Septoplasty Effectiveness Scale) should be obtained.

The nasal examination begins with external inspection. Careful attention is paid to the frontal view, examining for any asymmetry, particularly at the alar insertion. Flaccid facial paralysis may result in inferior and medial displacement of the ala on the paretic side.[6] Palpation of the middle third of the nose is helpful in determining the width of the internal valves. On the base view, the position of the columella, medial footplates, and caudal septum are all inspected. Again, alar base width and asymmetry are noted. Anterior rhinoscopy is performed next, with careful inspection of the septum, inferior turbinates, and internal and external valve area. Observation of the middle meatus and view of the middle turbinate should be noted. The shape and overall surface area of the external valve are observed. Lateral crura position and evidence of medial recurvature are also noted.

Returning to the base view, the dynamic examination is performed. The patient is asked to breathe normally through the nose while one

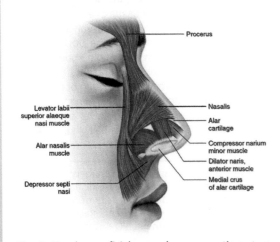

Fig. 1. Nasal superficial musculoaponeurotic system. (*From* Sugawara Y. (2020) Clinical Anatomy. In: A Practical Approach to Asian Rhinoplasty. Springer, Tokyo. 1-17.)

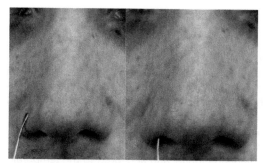

Fig. 2. The modified Cottle maneuver in the external valve batten position.

observes for dynamic nasal sidewall collapse and medial movement of the alar base. The modified Cottle maneuver is performed next in the external valve position or the area of most significant collapse. First, the lateral wall is merely stabilized in position, and normal inspiration is resumed while noting the patient's findings. Next, the lateral wall is lateralized approximately 1 mm and results are recorded (**Fig. 2**). The modified Cottle maneuver is then performed in the internal valve area (**Fig. 3**). The modified Cottle maneuvers are more specific for changes achieved with functional rhinoplasty grafts. Last, the Cottle maneuver, superolateral displacement of the patient's cheek, is performed, and the findings are recorded (**Fig. 4**). Typically, flaccid paralysis patients' symptoms are more significantly improved with this maneuver, as this addresses the inferomedial displacement of the alar base.

Two fundamental problems exist in patients with facial paralysis that lead to nasal obstruction. Patients with flaccid facial paralysis are more likely to have inferomedial displacement of the alar base of the paretic side (**Fig. 5**). Inferomedial displacement of the alar base of the paretic side may be observed in patients with incomplete paralysis if midfacial hypotonicity is present,[2] and this is an infrequent finding in patients with

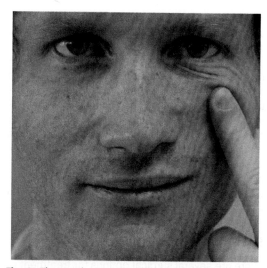

Fig. 4. The Cottle maneuver demonstrating superolateral displacement of the alar base.

nonflaccid paralysis, which is characterized by synkinesis and hypertonicity. External valve narrowing and dynamic valve collapse are also common findings in patients with facial paralysis because of loss of tone and function of the nasal sidewall and alar musculature.[3,4] Both of these issues should be explored and considered when treated these patients.

NONSURGICAL TREATMENT OPTIONS

It is important to discuss all treatment options for patients with nasal obstruction secondary to facial paralysis. Patients who are not surgical candidates or those who have only mild symptoms with minimal effect on quality of life may be amenable to

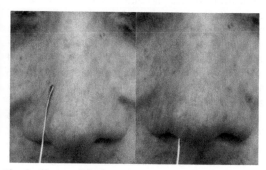

Fig. 3. The modified Cottle maneuver in the internal valve spreader position.

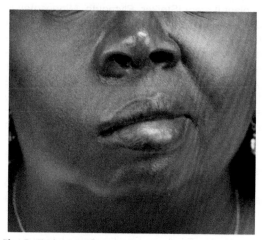

Fig. 5. Patient with right flaccid paralysis resulting in inferomedial displacement of the alar base resulting in nasal obstruction.

nonsurgical measures. If there is any evidence of underlying allergic or nonallergic rhinitis, intranasal steroids should be initiated. Vasomotor rhinitis, although no clear relationship exists in the literature, appears to occur more commonly on the side of paralysis in the authors' experience; ipratropium bromide nasal spray controls the symptoms well. Nasal dilators are options for nonsurgical patients. External adhesive dilators can be effective for patients with intermittent nasal obstruction or symptoms during specific activity, such as during exercising or sleeping. Internal dilators are also excellent options for patients with nighttime symptoms.

SURGICAL OPTIONS

There are several surgical options for treatment of nasal obstruction secondary to facial paralysis. Surgical decision making is largely based off the patient's symptoms and physical examination findings. Nasal valve augmentation is commonly performed during functional rhinoplasty with use of spreader grafts, flaring sutures, batten grafts, and lateral crural strut grafts. These techniques are very effective in patients with nasal valve insufficiency or collapse; however, they do not address one of the fundamental problems noted in patients with facial paralysis.[2]

For patients presenting with facial paralysis and nasal valve obstruction, nasal valve augmentation is frequently performed concurrently with facial reanimation procedures. There are specific scenarios when minimally invasive surgical intervention is preferred. For patients with adequate nasal valve caliber at rest but significant dynamic valve collapse on inspiration that is relieved by simply stabilizing the lateral wall, a bioabsorbable implant (Latera [Stryker, Plymouth, Minnesota]) is a reasonable option. This can be performed at the time of reanimation or in isolation. Bioabsorbable nasal sidewall implants have demonstrated significant NOSE score improvements 1 year postoperatively, but studies are not available for patients with facial paralysis.[9] More commonly, static nasal valve insufficiency is present concurrently with inferior-medial displacement of the ala, and obstruction is not relieved with only stabilization of the nasal sidewall. In these cases, more extensive nasal valve augmentation is required.

Several techniques have been described to address the inferomedial displacement of the ala frequently present in facial paralysis. Nasal valve suspension, first described by Paniello,[10] then simplified by Friedman,[11] redirects the lateral crura and sidewall in a superior-lateral direction. These techniques have been used in patients with facial

paralysis with significant improvement of symptoms.[4,12,13] Rose[14] first introduced a modification of nasal valve suspension with use of fascia lata. This technique was further described by Lindsay and colleagues[2] and demonstrated significant patient-reported quality-of-life improvement in patients with facial paralysis postoperatively. They describe making an incision within the alar crease and securing fascia lata to the sesamoid cartilage within the ala. The fascia is passed through a subcutaneous tunnel and anchored to the temporalis fascia, and this directs the alar base in a superolateral direction.

The authors' technique is similar to the fascia lata suspension mentioned above, with some subtle differences. This procedure makes use of an intranasal marginal incision rather than an external skin incision in the alar crease. Although an external incision in this location is well hidden, the resulting scar can be somewhat unpredictable and potentially visible.[15] The intranasal approach also allows for extended access to the lower and upper lateral cartilage of the lateral nasal wall to include these structures in the suspension along with the alar base if indicated based on patient examination findings.

The procedure is performed under general anesthesia. The distance from the ala to the helical root is measured. A fascia lata graft is then obtained from the lateral thigh measuring 2 cm longer than the measurement. The graft is 1 cm in width. A larger graft is harvested if other suspension procedures are planned. A vertical incision or stairstep horizontal incisions can be used to obtain the fascia. Once the graft is obtained, it is prestretched with 2 Kelly clamps and placed in saline for later use to limit postoperative relaxation of the graft.

A marginal incision is made and connected to a small back-cut anterior-inferiorly toward the piriform at the lateral extent of the incision (**Fig. 6**). The back-cut allows more room for tunneling from the alar base and access for suture placement from the alar fibrofatty tissue to the fascia lata graft. Dissection is performed over the lateral crura in a supra-perichondrial plane, and this can be extended over the scroll and upper lateral cartilage as needed depending on the area of maximal nasal valve collapse identified on preoperative examination. Once the lateral crura is adequately exposed, blunt dissection over the piriform aperture is performed. The piriform ligament can be transected at this point if lateralization of the alar base feels limited. A second incision is then made beginning within the hair-bearing skin of the temple. The true temporalis fascia is then exposed. The tendon passer is then tunneled

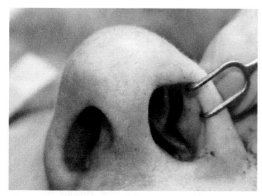

Fig. 6. Marginal incision with small back-cut for access to the pyriform.

from the margin incision to the temporal incision, and the prestretched fascia is pulled through (**Fig. 7**). The tendon passer crosses multiple planes as it begins deep at the level of the alar base and ends at the level of the temporalis fascia. The fascia is first secured to the lateral surface of the lateral crura with 4-0 PDS sutures. The suture passes through the lateral crura and vestibular mucosa while the knot is placed superficial to the fascia. Three to 4 sutures are typically placed into the areas of maximum valve collapse. The fascia is then pulled superolaterally and secured to the temporalis fascia with 3-0 Prolene sutures. The marginal incision is closed with 5-0 fast-gut sutures, and the temporal incision is closed with 5-0 Monocryl deep sutures and 5-0 Prolene skin sutures. Overcorrection by 2 to 3 mm is desired

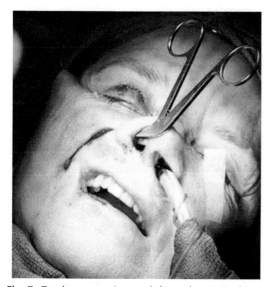

Fig. 7. Tendon passer inserted through marginal incision beginning deep in a supraperiosteal plane and ending through the temporal incision at the level of the temporalis fascia.

because some relaxation is anticipated in the postoperative period.

Postoperatively, a compression wrap is placed around the fascia lata donor site and kept in place for 1 week. A gentle compression dressing is placed around the temporal region and removed in 24 hours. Postoperative antibiotics are typically given for 1 week. The first postoperative visit occurs at 1 week for suture removal (**Fig. 8**).

COMPLICATIONS

Nasal valve suspension with fascia lata is a relatively straightforward and safe procedure. Autologous fascia lata has distinct advantages over synthetic graft material in facial suspension. Suspension with polytetrafluoroethylene has higher rates of infection, extrusion, and progressive stretching over time.[16,17] Acellular human dermis has lower infection rates but poor long-term outcomes because of stretch and absorption.[18] Complications of fascia lata harvest include scar, infection, hematoma, and pain with walking typically limited to less than 1 week.[19] In the authors' experience, complication rates of fascia lata harvest occur in less than 1% of cases.

The most common complication associated with nasal valve suspension with fascia lata in the authors' experience is relaxation over time. It is difficult to truly overwiden the alar base with this technique; thus, initial suspension should be rather tight. If relaxation occurs in months to years postoperatively, the temporal incision can be opened under local anesthetic, and the graft can be resuspended further posterior-superiorly to the temporalis fascia. Although absorbable PDS is used on the lateral crura suspension, the authors have not experienced dehiscence over time. The 6- to 9-month suture duration allows for significant scar formation between the fascia and the lateral crura. Other uncommon complications include infection, hematoma, and suture granuloma.

CURRENT EVIDENCE

Facial paralysis is a well-known significant cause of nasal obstruction first described by May and

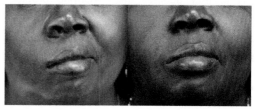

Fig. 8. Preoperative and 6-month postoperative visit after nasal valve sling.

colleagues.[20] Nasal valve suspension has been described to address the fundamental problem associated with nasal obstruction resulting from facial paralysis. Alex and Nguyen[13] first introduced nasal valve suture suspension techniques for treatment of patients with facial paralysis in 2004. Twelve patients were followed for 14 months postoperatively; 10 experienced significant improvement, whereas 2 patients reported moderate improvement of nasal breathing. Nuara and Mobley[12] performed nasal valve suspension on 9 patients with facial paralysis and demonstrated similar results; however, 2 patients experienced loss of suspension within 18 months, and 1 patient had an anchor site infection within 6 weeks. Soler and colleagues[4] performed a similar technique on 18 patients at the time of their initial facial nerve resection procedure. Two-year follow-up demonstrated significant improvement in NOSE scale scores compared with patients who did not undergo nasal valve suspension. No patients experienced loss of suspension or suture granuloma.

Nasal valve suspension with fascia lata in patients with facial paralysis has produced significant improvement in patient-reported quality of life.[2] Lindsay demonstrated this with 37 patients, while only 1 patient required fascia lata tightening postoperatively; however, long-term results with this technique are not available. The authors' technique avoids the alar crease incision, and in their experience, produces similar results.

SUMMARY

Nasal obstruction is a common, yet often overlooked, symptom associated with facial paralysis. Nasal valve-grafting is frequently used in traditional rhinoplasty for the treatment of internal and external valve collapse. Patients with flaccid paralysis have a fundamentally different mechanism causing nasal obstruction, which requires a different treatment approach. Although nasal sidewall insufficiency is present in these cases, inferomedial displacement of the ala results in a narrow external valve resulting in significant obstruction. Nonflaccid paralysis cases may be treated with traditional grafting techniques, but flaccid paralysis requires nasal valve sling to truly address the underlying problem. Several sling techniques have been described in the literature, which have demonstrated efficacious results. A slight modification of this technique uses fascia lata and eliminates the need for external facial scars by using marginal and temporal incisions for access. This technique produces similar results compared with other techniques and can be used in isolation or concurrently with other facial reanimation procedures.

CLINICS CARE POINTS

- Nasal valve obstruction commonly occurs in patients with facial paralysis resulting from inferomedial displacement of the ala and loss of function of the nasal dilator muscles.
- To address the fundamental problem in flaccid paralysis, nasal valve suspension should be performed to support the external valve and secure the alar base in a superolateral direction.
- Over-correction of 2-3 mm should be performed as some relaxation does occur in the postoperative period.
- Nasal valve suspension with fascia lata has demonstrated significant improvement in patient-reported quality of life for patients with flaccid facial paralysis.

DISCLOSURE

The authors have nothing to disclose.

REFERENCES

1. Hadlock TA, Greenfield LJ, Wernick-Robinson M, et al. Multimodality approach to management of the paralyzed face. Laryngoscope 2006;116(8): 1385–9.
2. Lindsay RW, Bhama P, Hohman M, et al. Prospective evaluation of quality-of-life improvement after correction of the alar base in the flaccidly paralyzed face. JAMA Facial Plast Surg 2015;17(2):108–12.
3. Bruintjes T, Olphen A, Hillen B, et al. A functional anatomic study of the relationship of the nasal cartilages and muscles to the nasal valve area. Laryngoscope 1998;108:1025–32.
4. Soler ZM, Rosenthal E, Wax MK. Immediate nasal valve reconstruction after facial nerve resection. Arch Facial Plast Surg 2008;10(5):312–5.
5. Mink PJ. Le nez comme voie respiratoire. Presse Otol Laryngol Belg 1903;2:481–96.
6. Bridger GP, Proctor DF. Maximum nasal inspiratory flow and nasal resistance. Ann Otol Rhinol Laryngol 1970;79(3):481–8.
7. Sugawara Y. Clinical anatomy. In: A practical approach to Asian rhinoplasty. Tokyo: Springer; 2020. p. 1–17.
8. Gassner HG, Sherris DA, Friedman O. 'Rhinology in Rhinoplasty' Ira D Papel. Facial plastic and reconstructive surgery. 4th edition. New York: Thieme Medical Publishers, Inc; 2016. p. 385–91.
9. Sidle DM, Stolovitzky P, Ow RA, et al. Twelve-month outcomes of a bioabsorbable implant for in-office

treatment of dynamic nasal valve collapse. Laryngoscope 2019. https://doi.org/10.1002/lary.28151.

10. Paniello RC. Nasal valve suspension. An effective treatment for nasal valve collapse. Arch Otolaryngol Head Neck Surg 1996;122:1342–6.

11. Friedman M, Ibrahim H, Lee G, et al. A simplified technique for airway correction at the nasal valve area. Otolaryngol Head Neck Surg 2004;131:519–24.

12. Nuara M, Mobley S. Nasal valve suspension revisited. Laryngoscope 2007;117(2):2100–6.

13. Alex JC, Nguyen DB. Multivectored suture suspension: a minimally invasive technique for reanimation of the paralyzed face. Arch Facial Plast Surg 2004; 6:197–201.

14. Rose EH. Autogenous fascia lata grafts: clinical applications in reanimation of the totally or partially paralyzed face. Plast Reconstr Surg 2005;116(1): 20–32.

15. Kridel RW, Castellano RD. A simplified approach to alar base reduction: a review of 124 patients over 20 years. Arch Facial Plast Surg 2005;7(2):81–93.

16. BielMA. GORE-TEX graft midfacial suspension and upper eyelid gold-weight implantation in rehabilitation of the paralyzed face. Laryngoscope 1995; 105(8, pt 1):876–9.

17. Constantinides M, Galli SK, Miller PJ. Complications of static facial suspensions with expanded polytetrafluoroethylene (ePTFE). Laryngoscope 2001; 111(12):2114–21.

18. Fisher E, Frodel JL. Facial suspension with acellular human dermal allograft. Arch Facial Plast Surg 1999;1(3):195–9.

19. Wheatcroft SM, Vardy SJ, Tyers AG. Complications of fascia lata harvesting for ptosis surgery. Br J Ophthalmol 1997;81(7):581–3.

20. May M, West JW, Hinderer KH. Nasal obstruction from facial palsy. Arch Otolaryngol 1977;103(7): 389–91.

Eyelid Coupling Using a Modified Tarsoconjunctival Flap in Facial Paralysis

Raj D. Dedhia, MD[a], Taha Z. Shipchandler, MD[b],
Travis T. Tollefson, MD, MPH[c],*

KEYWORDS

- Eyelid coupling • Tarsoconjunctival flap • Facial paralysis • Paralytic ectropion • Canthoplasty
- Canthopexy • Lagophthalmos

KEY POINTS

- Eyelid coupling using the modified tarsoconjunctival flap is an effective treatment for paralytic ectropion.
- Eyelid position and quality of life can be improved in patients with flaccid facial paralysis using these eyelid coupling procedures.
- The modified tarsoconjunctival flap can obscure the lateral visual field by coupling the eyelids, but without distortion of the canthal angle and eyelid margin.
- The procedure is often coupled with a lateral canthoplasty or canthopexy to address horizontal laxity of the lower eyelid.
- Collecting standardized outcome measures will help establish the ideal treatment paradigm of paralytic eyelid malposition.

INTRODUCTION

The primary function of the eyelids is to maintain ocular health and protection. The natural blink mechanism provides the eye with a protective tear film, prevents corneal desiccation and injury, and facilitates the flow of tears.[1] Eyelid function relies on a complex array of muscles that retract and elevate in coordinated fashion. Patients with facial paralysis lose that coordinated function and can present with profound ocular sequelae. Most notable is the loss of sphincter function of the orbicularis oculi muscle.[2]

In the paralyzed face, loss of orbicularis oculi function results in unopposed action of the upper-eyelid retractors (levator palpebrae superioris and Mullers muscle) and lower-eyelid retractors (inferior tarsal muscle).[1] This subsequently leads to an increase in palpebral fissure height and lagophthalmos, which put the eye at risk for complications from exposure. Other factors, such as age, scarring, or radiation therapy, can affect eyelid function and exacerbate the functional impairment.[3] Impaired blink from dynamic dysfunction of the eyelids results in poor tear film distribution and clearance through the lacrimal pump.[4] This

Conflicts of Interest: none.
[a] Department of Otolaryngology–Head and Neck Surgery, University of Tennessee Health Science Center, Memphis, TN, USA; [b] Department of Otolaryngology–Head and Neck Surgery, Indiana University School of Medicine, 340 West 10th Street, Indianapolis, IN 46202, USA; [c] Department of Otolaryngology–Head and Neck Surgery, University of California, Davis, 2521 Stockton Boulevard, Suite 7200, Sacramento, CA, USA
* Corresponding author.
E-mail address: tttollefson@ucdavis.edu

facialplastic.theclinics.com

may manifest in epiphora, presence of a tear lake, and dryness from ineffective ocular lubrication. Corneal protection by limiting lagophthalmos is important to prevent exposure keratopathy.[5] Lower-eyelid malposition is a major contributor to ocular sequalae of facial paralysis and is characterized by paralytic ectropion and retraction. The ectropion demonstrates eyelid eversion, whereas retraction is seen as downward gravitational pull on the eyelid (**Fig. 1**A).

The goals of treating the paralyzed eyelid complex are to protect the cornea and restore facial symmetry. Initial management frequently includes a moisture chamber and ocular lubrication to protect the cornea. Further intervention typically involves a combined approach to the upper and lower eyelids. For patients with suspected transient facial paresis, options include eyelid taping, temporary tarsorrhaphy, and induction of protective upper-eyelid ptosis with botulinum toxin. For chronic facial paralysis, upper-eyelid loading aids the retracted eyelid and helps prevent lagophthalmos. To address lower-eyelid malposition, a spectrum of techniques has been described that (1) shorten and/or tighten the lower eyelid, (2) suspend the lower eyelid, (3) support the middle lamella, (4) release retractors of the lower eyelid, or (5) connect the lower and upper eyelids.[1,6–12]

For chronic, flaccid facial paralysis, early postoperative success is often marred by inadequate eyelid position over time. The need for imporved long-term outcomes explains the continued pursuit of novel and modified eyelid procedures to treat paralytic ectropion. The authors of this article have favored an eyelid-coupling procedure using the modified tarsoconjunctival flap to correct paralytic ectropion.[6,7] The procedure is often used in conjunction with a lateral strip canthoplasty to address horizontal laxity. The modified tarsoconjunctival flap couples and balances the effect of the previously unopposed upper- and lower-eyelid retractors, thereby improving eyelid malposition and lagophthalmos. The flap also provides a vertical vector of support to the lower eyelid that is not provided by the lateral strip canthoplasty alone. Finally, the coupling provides dynamic benefit by allowing the upper-eyelid retractors to raise the lower eyelid (and vice versa), improving tear film distribution (eg, the squeegee effect). The modified tarsoconjunctival flap has advantages over traditional eyelid coupling surgery (eg, tarsorrhaphy), as it does create less distortion than the canthal angle and eyelid and is easily reversible (see **Fig. 1**B). Here, the authors describe their surgical technique and discuss patient outcomes.

SURGICAL TECHNIQUE

Lateral eyelid coupling is accomplished by insetting an upper-eyelid tarsoconjunctival flap into the lower eyelid. This procedure is frequently combined with either a lateral tarsal strip *canthoplasty* or a *canthopexy* with lateral retinacular suspension to address horizontal laxity. The tarsal strip canthoplasty differs from a canthopexy by including a through-and-through canthotomy/cantholysis. The canthopexy is achieved by using a lateral canthal skin incision to approach the inferior limb of the lateral canthal tendon, which is suspended upward and laterally with a suture to the medial aspect of the lateral orbital wall.

There are 4 main steps to this procedure:

(1) Create a tarsal strip or expose the lateral retinacular suspension

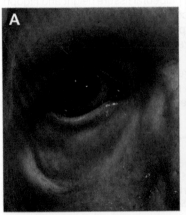
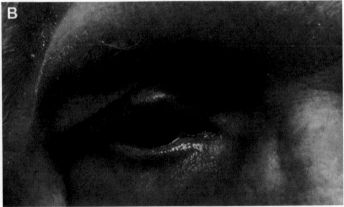

Fig. 1. (*A*) Paralytic ectropion and retraction of the right lower eyelid. There is punctal eversion, a tear lake, and conjunctival injection from exposure. (*B*) After eyelid coupling with a modified tarsoconjunctival flap, there is improvement in eyelid position.

(2) Elevate a superiorly based tarsoconjunctival flap from the upper eyelid

(3) Inset tarsoconjunctival flap into the lower eyelid

(4) Suspend the lateral canthal tendon to the lateral orbit (canthoplasty or canthopexy)

In step 1, the lateral canthotomy and inferior cantholysis are performed. Once the lower eyelid is free from its attachment to Whitnall tubercle, the lateral canthal tendon is then prepared by denuding the lateral skin and conjunctiva. A full-thickness excision of the lateral canthal tendon is performed to the degree needed to correct lower-eyelid laxity. The canthoplasty or cantho-pexy suture is parachuted in horizontal mattress fashion with either a 5-0 Polydiaxanone or 5-0 Poly(ethylene terephthalate) suture through the lateral canthal tendon and lateral orbital rim periosteum (superior and posterior to Whitnall tubercle). The suture is placed at this time, as it is more difficult to place once the tarsoconjunctival flap has been inset. This suture suspension of the lateral canthus is not tied until step 4.

In step 2, the upper eyelid is inverted over a DesMarres retractor using a 4-0 silk traction suture placed through the gray line. Hydrodissection with local anesthetic of the upper-eyelid tarsoconjunctival flap assists with flap elevation. The superiorly based flap is planned at the lateral aspect of the upper eyelid. The flap is designed to be 3 to 8 mm wide (adjustable to severity of eyelid laxity and snap test result) and 4 mm tall and includes the superior 1 to 2 mm of the tarsal plate (**Fig. 2**).

In step 3, an incision is made at the gray line at the lateral aspect of the lower eyelid, and a small sliver of lid margin is denuded to create a pocket to inset the tarsoconjunctival flap. The flap is then elevated and brought down in the usual

fashion for a modified Hughes tarsoconjunctival flap (**Fig. 3**) and sutured into the pocket with 4-0 polygalactin suture in interrupted fashion (**Fig. 4**). To prevent ocular injury or irritation, it is key to place the knots facing away from sclera.

In step 4, the canthoplasty or canthopexy suture placed in step 1 is then tied down. The lateral canthal angle can be re-created with a 6-0 fast-absorbing gut suture, which is secured under the 6-0 silk sutures used for the skin layer of the canthotomy/canthopexy closure. Before the skin closure, a deep layer with interrupted 5-0 Poliglecaprone sutures is used to approximate the wound edges.

DISCUSSION

There is no absolutely effective treatment for the eyelid manifestations of facial paralysis for all patients. The surgical techniques used are varied based on the severity of the paralysis, senile changes to the eyelids, and anatomic variations (eg, negative vector midface position). Comparing the reported techniques has been difficult because of dogma and a lack of uniform outcome measures reported in the literature.

Growing experience with the modified tarsoconjunctival flap is evident in the literature. Tao and colleagues[13] published the largest series (n = 110) of patients undergoing tarsoconjunctival flaps for paralytic ectropion.[13] The procedure was combined with a lateral canthoplasty (n = 45) when horizontal laxity was identified. In their cohort, lagophthalmos, exposure keratopathy, and eyelid retraction improved in all cases. The investigators describe an additional dynamic benefit, especially in patients with a strong Bell reflex, as the lower eyelid elevated during upward movement of the eye. It is postulated that this finding may be secondary to the flap's attachments to the fornix. Although these results favor the use of this technique, the lack of reported facial

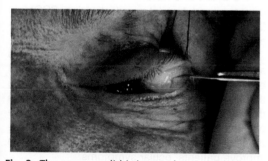

Fig. 2. The upper eyelid is inverted over a DesMarres retractor using a 4-0 silk traction suture placed through the gray line. The superiorly based tarsoconjunctival flap is planned at the lateral aspect of the upper eyelid and designed to be 3 to 6 mm wide, 4 mm tall, and includes the superior 1 to 2 mm of the tarsal plate.

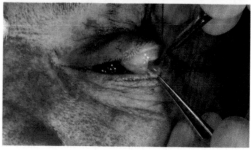

Fig. 3. The flap is elevated, leaving only the conjunctiva attached, and brought down in the usual fashion for a modified Hughes tarsoconjunctival flap.

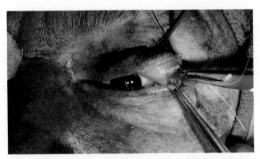

Fig. 4. After a recipient pocket is created at the gray line of the lower eyelid, the tarsoconjunctival flap is inset and sutured into the pocket with 4-0 polygalactin suture in interrupted fashion.

paralysis severity and quantifiable patient-reported outcome measures (PROM) prevent generalized application to facial paralysis patients.

The Facial Clinimetric Evaluation (FaCE) instrument is a patient-reported quality-of-life metric that scores facial movement, facial comfort, oral function, eye comfort, lacrimal control, and social function.[14] Dedhia and colleagues[7] reported their modified tarsoconjunctival flap outcomes in patients with flaccid facial paralysis using the FaCE instrument and ectropion grading scale (EGS).[15] The outcomes were stratified by those that received periorbital or midface radiation therapy. Patients who had received radiation therapy demonstrated improvement in eye comfort and lacrimal control subdomain scores of the FaCE instrument, whereas no difference was seen in

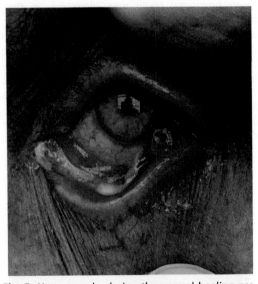

Fig. 5. Uncommonly, during the normal healing process, a frond of granulation will form around the tarsoconjunctival flap. Pyogenic granuloma, such as these, are temporary and amenable to ophthalmologic ointment, such as dexamethasone/neomycin sulfate/polymyxin B sulfate.

patients who had not undergone radiation therapy; all patients had improved eyelid position as graded by the EGS. Outcomes from future studies on paralytic ectropion that report these standardized metrics (ie, FaCE scale and EGS) can be used to compare efficacy of treatment and help elucidate which procedures are optimal for a given patient.

Complications with the tarsoconjunctival flap are rare. The authors' experience is consistent with that which has been previously reported by Tao and colleagues,[13] who reported a flap dehiscence rate of 2.6%, which was easily treated with repeat suturing; pyogenic granuloma rate of 4.5%, which required excision; and loss of peripheral vision rate of 6.4%, which was treated with partial flap division under local anesthesia. In the authors' experience, around 10% of cases develop a temporary granulation tissue, consistent with pyogenic granuloma (**Fig. 5**). Patients will complain of dried crusting of the lateral canthal region and are amenable to antibiotic/steroid ointments or drops. Most likely, these are normal healing responses to the polygalactin sutures used for the closure.

In the past several years, many surgical treatment options to address the eyelids in facial paralysis have been described (eg, paralytic ectropion repair). These options include eyelid coupling,[7] orbicularis oculi turnover procedures,[9] eyelid reanimation with a modified temporalis muscle flap,[10] bipedicled orbicularis oculi myocutaneous flap,[11] lower-eyelid retractor recession, and lateral horn lysis.[12] In these studies, margin to reflex distance-2, lower-eyelid height, EGS, and FaCE instrument metrics were used to report outcomes. In addition, the FaCE scale was used in recent studies to analyze how gracilis free flap,[16] temporalis transposition,[16] and hypoglossal nerve jump graft to report outcomes,[17] including their effect on the eyelid and lacrimal subdomains. Although the increased trend toward studying PROM in facial paralysis will help elucidate optimal treatment, more work is needed.

Larger studies using unified outcome metrics are needed to identify which techniques are the best in different patient populations. In addition, the effect of other facial reanimation techniques that provide periocular innervation or midface support need to be studied in a similar fashion to understand how these combined techniques can improve patients' ocular symptoms.

SUMMARY

Eyelid coupling using the modified tarsoconjunctival flap is an effective treatment to improve eyelid closure in patients with facial paralysis. Improved eyelid position and patient outcomes with validated quality-of-life metrics have been demonstrated using this technique. Further studies with standardized outcome measures are needed to elucidate the optimal periocular treatment for patients with facial paralysis.

DISCLOSURES

None.

REFERENCES

1. Joseph SS, Joseph AW, Douglas RS, et al. Periocular reconstruction in patients with facial paralysis. Otolaryngol Clin North Am 2016;49(2):475–87.

2. Sibony PA, Evinger C, Manning KA. Eyelid movements in facial paralysis. Arch Ophthalmol 1991; 109(11):1555–61.

3. Bedran EG, Pereira MV, Bernardes TF. Ectropion. Semin Ophthalmol 2010;25(3):59–65.

4. Bergeron CM, Moe KS. The evaluation and treatment of lower eyelid paralysis. Facial Plast Surg 2008;24(2):231–41.

5. Chang L, Olver J. A useful augmented lateral tarsal strip tarsorrhaphy for paralytic ectropion. Ophthalmology 2006;113(1):84–91.

6. Sufyan AS, Lee HB, Shah H, et al. Single-stage repair of paralytic ectropion using a novel modification of the tarsoconjunctival flap. JAMA Facial Plast Surg 2014;16(2):151–2.

7. Dedhia R, Hsieh TY, Chin O, et al. Outcomes from lateral eyelid coupling for facial paralysis using the modified tarsoconjunctival flap. JAMA Facial Plast Surg 2018;20(5):381–6.

8. Kwon KY, Jang SY, Yoon JS. Long-term outcome of combined lateral tarsal strip with temporal permanent tarsorrhaphy for correction of paralytic ectropion caused by facial nerve palsy. J Craniofac Surg 2015;26(5):e409–12.

9. Azuma R, Aoki S, Aizawa T, et al. The vertical orbicularis oculi muscle turn-over procedure for the correction of paralytic ectropion of the lower eyelid. Arch Plast Surg 2018;45(2):135–9.

10. Evrenos MK, Bali ZU, Yaman M, et al. Modified temporalis muscle flap for eyelid reanimation. J Craniofac Surg 2018;29(7):e649–54.

11. Fleischman GM, Thorp BD, Shockley WW, et al. The bipedicled orbicularis oculi myocutaneous flap for the repair of paralytic ectropion. JAMA Facial Plast Surg 2019;21(2):169–71.

12. Tan P, Wong J, Siah WF, et al. Outcomes of lower eyelid retractor recession and lateral horn lysis in lower eyelid elevation for facial nerve palsy. Eye (Lond) 2018;32(2):338–44.

13. Tao JP, Vemuri S, Patel AD, et al. Lateral tarsoconjunctival onlay flap lower eyelid suspension in facial nerve paresis. Ophthal Plast Reconstr Surg 2014; 30(4):342–5.

14. Kahn JB, Gliklich RE, Boyev KP, et al. Validation of a patient-graded instrument for facial nerve paralysis: the FaCE scale. Laryngoscope 2001;111(3):387–98.

15. Moe KS, Linder T. The lateral transorbital canthopexy for correction and prevention of ectropion: report of a procedure, grading system, and outcome study. Arch Facial Plast Surg 2000;2(1):9–15.

16. Van veen MM, Dijkstra PU, Le coultre S, et al. Gracilis transplantation and temporalis transposition in long-standing facial palsy in adults: patient-reported and aesthetic outcomes. J Craniomaxillofac Surg 2018; 46(12):2144–9.

17. Volk GF, Geitner M, Geißler K, et al. Functional outcome and quality of life after hypoglossal-facial jump nerve suture. Front Surg 2020;7:11.

Modified Selective Neurectomy
A New Paradigm in the Management of Facial Palsy with Synkinesis

Babak Azizzadeh, MD, Nikolaus Hjelm, MD*

KEYWORDS

- Modified selective neurectomy • Synkinesis • Facial paralysis • Smile

KEY POINTS

- There are several techniques and approaches to treat facial synkinesis.
- Modified selective neurectomy is the only treatment of synkinesis that preserves the natural neural pathway while maintaining long-lasting results.
- The patient regains their natural smile without sacrificing cosmesis.
- The depressor anguli oris, platysma, buccinator, and mentalis are the synkinetic muscles that prevent a natural smile.

INTRODUCTION

Postfacial paralysis with synkinesis presents with a multitude of facial movement disorders.[1–4] In addition to smile dysfunction, patients can present with unintentional motion of the face when a voluntary motion is attempted. The most common unintentional movements are that of the oral commissure with eye closure (oculo-oral) and eye closure with talking or smiling (oro-ocular). Although the cause of synkinesis is poorly understood, aberrant nerve regeneration has been considered as the most likely cause. Aberrant regeneration describes the regrowth of a motor nerve following nerve injury, producing multiple terminal axons that innervate nonnative muscle groups.[5,6] The physical manifestations of synkinesis has not been clearly elucidated. However, recent studies have confirmed that the smile dysfunction is likely secondary to overactivity of counterproductive muscles that cause downward and lateral oral excursion such as the depressor anguli oris, platysma, buccinator, mentalis, and orbicularis oris.[1–22] These counteractive muscles concurrently contract with variable strength leading to synkinesis. In addition to smile dysfunction, this involuntary and variable muscular contraction can also cause the patient to experience oral incompetence.

Initial treatment of postparalytic synkinesis has been focused on chemodenervation with botulinum toxin type A (BTA) with or without concurrent physical therapy.[7–9] This treatment approach has produced objective and subjective results, including improved facial symmetry, reduced involuntary muscle contractions, and enhanced quality of life.[7] The role of physical therapy should not be understated; neuromuscular retraining with BTA injections can lead to persistent improvement in synkinesis and imbalance after the chemodenervation wears off.[8]

Static and dynamic surgical options have been used extensively to treat patients with facial nerve disorders to improve oral competence and increase oral commissure excursion. Of note, orthodromic temporalis tendon transfer, gracilis functional free muscle transfer, and masseteric and/or hypoglossal to facial nerve transfer have found success and are the widely used methods of treatment.[10–19] Although the indications for

The Facial Paralysis Institute, 9401 Wilshire Boulevard, Suite 650, Beverly Hills, CA 90212, USA
* Corresponding author.
E-mail address: nshjelm@gmail.com

Facial Plast Surg Clin N Am 29 (2021) 453–457
https://doi.org/10.1016/j.fsc.2021.03.005
1064-7406/21/© 2021 Elsevier Inc. All rights reserved.

each procedure depend on the surgeon's preference as well as the cause and timing of the facial palsy, all of these procedures were developed to address complete flaccid paralysis.

Although the existing dynamic reanimation options have clearly improved patient outcomes over the past 2 decades, none addresses the underlying cause of synkinesis. Furthermore, utilization of the motor nucleus of the trigeminal nerve (temporalis tendon transfer and masseteric-facial nerve transfer) as the driving force of smile mechanism results in a nonspontaneous mimetic movement. Dynamic treatment methods such as gracilis muscle free flaps and temporalis tendon transfers further distance the patient from their natural smile by bypassing the native muscles of facial expression for oral commissure elevation. If cross-face nerve grafts are used, the muscles of facial expression are subject to different motor nuclei and variable overall axonal innervation, causing variable strength and timing of contraction. To improve on current treatment methods, the senior author (BA) has shifted the paradigm in the management of smile dysfunction in facial palsy with synkinesis by developing a denervation technique called "modified selective neurectomy" that addresses the underlying cause of smile synkinesis, thereby achieving long-term natural and spontaneous outcome.[2-4,14] This operation results in the most natural treatment of synkinesis, as it preserves the entire neural pathway from the facial motor nucleus in the pons to the muscle fibers. By preserving the innate efferent neural pathway, modified selective neurectomy enables patients to maintain their natural spontaneous smile.

Selective surgical denervation of synkinetic muscles is particularly helpful around the mouth where there is a convergence of muscles around the oral commissure at the modiolus as well as in the upper and lower lip. The synkinetic "tug of war" between these muscles causes smile dysfunction in affected patients. Therefore, reducing muscles that negatively affect the smile at the nerve level can allow the appropriate muscles to activate unencumbered. Chemodenervation in this area has yielded poor smile outcomes because the muscles are in such close proximity that it is very difficult to selectively reduce the activity of counterproductive muscles.

Technical details used in the modified selective neurectomy have resulted in outcomes that are long term. Permanent denervation is completed by excising segments of aberrant facial nerve branches and placing titanium clips to the nerve ends to prevent regrowth.[3] In addition to studies using blinded observers validating long-term

results, patients undergoing modified selective neurectomy were also found to have decreased BTA requirements over time.[2,4,20] Previous denervation techniques to address ocular synkinesis did not yield long-term results likely due to the fact that a singular muscle (orbicularis oculi) is responsible for narrowing eyelid aperture.[21,22] There are no counteractive muscles that cause that, and and extensive denervation would be required to avoid recurrence.

SURGICAL PROCEDURE

Preparation/Incision
- Patient is transorally intubated and placed under general anesthesia without paralytics.
- A standard retrotragal rhytidectomy incision is planned.
- The incision and subcutaneous plane of the face is injected with 1:100,000 epinephrine. Lidocaine is not recommended as to avoid inadvertent decrease of neural activity.
- Facial nerve monitoring electrodes are placed in the periorbital and perioral regions.
- Incision is made with a #15 blade down to the subcutaneous layer.

Dissection
- Starting at the temporal hair tuft, subcutaneous dissection is extended medially for 4 to 6 cm from the incision.
- An incision is then made in the superficial musculoaponeurotic system (SMAS) and platysma and in an oblique vector from the lateral zygomatic arch to the cervical region passing through the angle of the mandible.
- The SMAS and platysma are elevated as a single flap for 3 to 6 cm.
- Dissection is carried out deep to the masseteric and subplatysmal fascia in order to identify the branches of the facial nerve as they exit the parotid capsule (**Fig. 1**).

Nerve Identification
- All visible branches of the zygomatic, buccal, marginal mandibular, and cervical divisions of the facial nerve are identified and carefully dissected.
- The connections between the zygomatic and buccal branches are isolated as well as side branches of the cervical branches, as they enter the underbelly of the platysma.
- The nerve branches are then stimulated at 0.5 to 2.0 mA to evaluate the elicited movement.
- Nerve branches that cause platysmal tightening or downward and lateral excursion of the oral commissure are isolated (**Fig. 2**).
- Video evaluation of the movement is recorded.

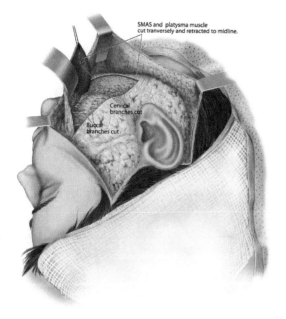

Fig. 1. Surgical approach for modified selective neurectomy. Entering the deep plane allows for optimal exposure to identify and transect/preserve facial nerve branches as they exit the parotid capsule. (*Courtesy of* Dr. Azizzadeh, Facial Paralysis Institute.)

- Titanium clips are placed on the most proximal and distal portion of the dissected nerve, and 0.5 to 4.0 cm of intervening nerve is resected.
- The zygomatic branches that purely elevate the oral commissure and the marginal mandibular branch that stimulates the depressor labii inferioris are carefully preserved.

- One or two branches that close the lips are preserved to maintain oral competence.
- A platysma myotomy is performed below the identified marginal mandibular nerve.
- Symmetric facial repositioning and autologous fat grafting as described by Hjelm and Azizzadeh in 2020 may be performed as needed to improve soft tissue asymmetry at rest (**Fig. 3**).[20]

Closure

- SMAS is redraped and sutured into the prior natural position.
- Drains are placed over the SMAS and under the skin flap.
- Incision line is redraped and sutured into the prior natural position.
- Suction is applied to drains to confirm that there are no leaks.
- Pressure dressing is typically not used.

COMPLICATIONS AND POSTOPERATIVE COURSE

Patients are discharged the same day and typically return to work within 10 days. BTA for bilateral periorbital regions may be injected beginning 1 week postoperatively as needed.[2] Articulation variances and ocular synkinesis typically do not improve with modified selective neurectomy. Neuromuscular retraining begins 1 month postoperatively with the instruction of trained facial nerve physical therapists. Final outcomes have been observed between 6 months and 1 year.[2] Observed complications by the senior author (BA) consist of hematoma, seroma, and temporary oral incompetence.[2,3] No other major complications have been encountered by the senior author. A subset of patients has required revision surgery when synkinesis has not resolved to

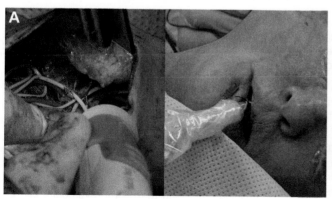
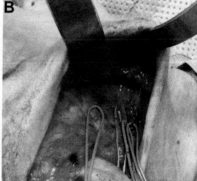

Fig. 2. (*A*) Nerve branches that cause platysmal tightening or downward and lateral excursion of the oral commissure are identified by electrical stimulation. (*B*) These branches are then isolated and tagged with vessel loops for resection. (*Courtesy of* Dr. Azizzadeh, Facial Paralysis Institute.)

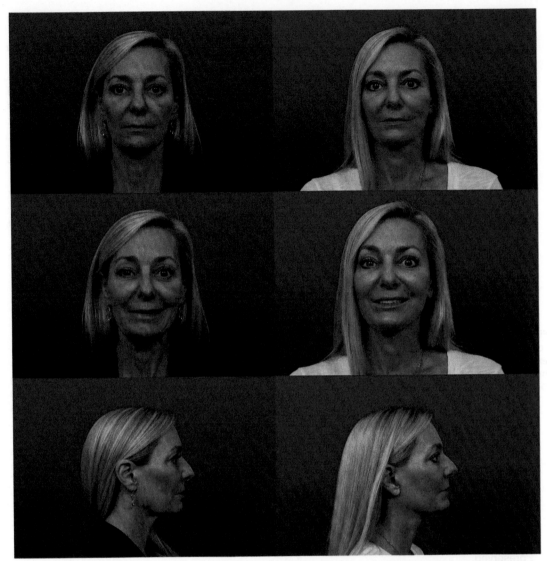

Fig. 3. Preoperative (left) and 1-month postoperative (right) photographs of a patient following modified selective neurectomy with symmetric facial repositioning. The postoperative photographs show improved symmetry, smile, and decreased synkinesis. (*Courtesy of* Dr. Azizzadeh, Facial Paralysis Institute.)

surgeon and/or patient satisfaction. In these patients, the senior author (BA) has noted adequate resolution of synkinesis following revision modified selective neurectomy. Revision surgery should be considered after 1 year.

SUMMARY

All patients with postparalytic paralysis are at risk of developing synkinesis. Causes are diverse; however, from the senior author's (BA) experience, patients with synkinesis most often recovered from Bells palsy or Ramsay Hunt syndrome. A subset of patients with facial palsy after temporal bone fracture and acoustic neuroma resection

may also develop synkinesis. When the synkinesis causes smile dysfunction, there are several treatment modalities available per physician preference. Modified selective neurectomy of the facial nerve is offered to patients who have nonprogressive synkinesis, active zygomatic major/minor muscles, and intact distal branches of the facial nerve. Exclusionary criteria consist of complete flaccid paralysis and malignancy. Studies have shown that in the correctly selected patient, modified selective neurectomy is effective in accomplishing a long-term improvement in the spontaneous smile mechanism in patients with synkinesis.

CLINICS CARE POINTS

- Patient selection is first and foremost critical. Patients must have stable synkinesis over time, active zygomatic major/minor muscles, and intact distal branches of the facial nerve. Exclusionary criteria consist of complete flaccid paralysis and malignancy.

- Patient expectations and goals must be discussed preoperatively.

- Patients must not be paralyzed during surgery, and it is advised that the incision line is not injected with lidocaine hydrochloride as to prevent inadvertent paresis of the facial nerve.

- Nerve monitoring is imperative for identifying synkinetic nerve fibers.

- Prior study has shown that patients had the best results when, on average, 6.7 nerves were excised.

- Postoperatively, patients have experienced subjective benefits with neuromuscular retraining by trained facial nerve physical therapists.

DISCLOSURE

Dr. Azizzadeh gets royalties from Elsevier and Quality Medical Publishing.

REFERENCES

1. Crumley RL. Mechanisms of synkinesis. Laryngoscope 1979;89(11):1847–54.
2. Azizzadeh B, Irvine LE, Diels JO, et al. Modified Selective Neurectomy for the Treatment of Post–Facial Paralysis Synkinesis. Plast Reconstr Surg 2019; 143(5):1483–96.
3. Hjelm N, Azizzadeh B. Modified Selective Neurectomy with Symmetrical Facial Repositioning. Facial Plast Surg Aesthet Med 2020;22(1):57–60.
4. Azizzadeh B, Frisenda JL. Surgical Management of Postparalysis Facial Palsy and Synkinesis. Otolaryngol Clin Oto North Am 2018;51(6):1169–78.
5. Husseman J, Mehta RP. Management of synkinesis. Facial Plast Surg 2008;24(2):242–9.
6. Montserrat L, Benito M. Facial synkinesis and aberrant regeneration of facial nerve. In: Jankovic J, Tolos E, editors. Advances in neurology. New York: Raven Press; 1988. p. 211–24.
7. Shinn JR, Nwabueze NN, Du L, et al. Treatment Patterns and Outcomes in Botulinum Therapy for Patients With Facial Synkinesis. JAMA Facial Plast Surg 2019;21(3):244–51.
8. Cabin JA, Massry GG, Azizzadeh B. Botulinum toxin in the management of facial paralysis. Curr Opin Otolaryngol Head Neck Surg 2015;23(4):272–80.
9. Borodic G, Bartley M, Slattery W, et al. Botulinum toxin for aberrant facial nerve regeneration: double-blind, placebo-controlled trial using subjective endpoints. Plast Reconstr Surg 2005;116(1): 36–43.
10. Burkhalter WE. Early tendon transfer in upper extremity peripheral nerve injury. Clin Orthop Relat Res 1974;104:68–79.
11. Boahene KD. Temporalis Muscle Tendon Unit Transfer for Smile Restoration After Facial Paralysis. Facial Plast Surg Clin North Am 2016;24(1):37–45.
12. Boahene KD, Farrag TY, Ishii L, et al. Minimally invasive temporalis tendon transposition. Arch Facial Plast Surg 2011;13(1):8–13.
13. Jowett N, Hadlock TA. Free Gracilis Transfer and Static Facial Suspension for Midfacial Reanimation in Long-Standing Flaccid Facial Palsy. Otolaryngol Clin North Am 2018;51(6):1129–39.
14. Vincent AG, Bevans SE, Robitschek JM, et al. Masseteric-to-Facial Nerve Transfer and Selective Neurectomy for Rehabilitation of the Synkinetic Smile. JAMA Facial Plast Surg 2019;21(6):504–10.
15. Klebuc MJ. Facial reanimation using the masseter-to-facial nerve transfer. Plast Reconstr Surg 2011; 127:1909.
16. Gousheh J, Arasteh E. Treatment of facial paralysis: dynamic reanimation of spontaneous facial expression-apropos of 655 patients. Plast Reconstr Surg 2011;128(6):693e–703e.
17. Van de Graaf RC, IJpma FF, Nicolai JP. Facial reanimation by means of the hypoglossal nerve: anatomic comparison of different techniques. Neurosurgery 2008;63(4):E820.
18. Zhang S, Hembd A, Ching CW, et al. Early masseter to facial nerve transfer may improve smile excursion in facial paralysis. Plast Reconstr Surg Glob Open 2018;6(11):e2023.
19. Hohman MH, Hadlock TA. Etiology, diagnosis, and management of facial palsy: 2000 patients at a facial nerve center. Laryngoscope 2014;124(7):E283–93.
20. Hjelm N, Crippen M, Azizzadeh B. Long-Term Changes in the Treatment Pattern of Botulinum Toxin A injections for post-facial paralysis synkinesis following modified selective neurectomy. Facial Plast Surg Aesthet Med 2020. https://doi.org/10.1089/fpsam.2020.0240.
21. Hohman MH, Lee LN, Hadlock TA. Two-step highly selective neurectomy for refractory periocular synkinesis. Laryngoscope 2013;123:1385–8.
22. Van Veen MM, Dusseldorp JR, Hadlock TA. Long-term outcome of selective neurectomy for refractory periocular synkinesis. Laryngoscope 2018;128(10): 2291–5.

Corneal and Facial Sensory Neurotization in Trigeminal Anesthesia

Nate Jowett, MD[a],*, Roberto Pineda II, MD[b]

KEYWORDS

- Corneal disease • Nerve regeneration • Trigeminal nerve • Keratopathy • Trigeminal anesthesia
- Facial anesthesia • Trigeminal trophic syndrome

KEY POINTS

- Trigeminal anesthesia may yield blindness and facial disfigurement.
- The pathophysiology of the tissue insult in trigeminal anesthesia comprises a loss of protective sensory feedback and loss of afferent neural trophic support.
- Mounting evidence supports a role for sensory nerve transfers in the management of trigeminal anesthesia.

INTRODUCTION

The somatosensory system is highly conserved in evolution.[1] Touch is the first sensation to develop in humans[2] and plays a pivotal role in normal growth and development.[3] A congenital absence of or insult to the somatosensory fibers of the trigeminal nerve yields facial anesthesia. Trigeminal neuropathy may arise from viral or bacterial infection (eg, herpes zoster, leprosy, syphilis), neuroinflammatory disorders (eg, multiple sclerosis, sarcoidosis), rheumatologic disorders (eg, systemic lupus erythematosus, vasculitis), cerebrovascular arteriovenous malformations and infarcts, skull base tumors and their extirpation (eg, meningiomas, schwannomas), and trigeminal ganglion ablation for therapeutic management of trigeminal neuralgia. Beyond its potential role in the growth and development and sense of self, facial sensation is necessary for the protection and normal function of the ocular surface and facial soft tissues. Trigeminal anesthesia may cause corneal blindness, functional impairment with the oral phase of deglutition, and facial disfigurement (**Fig. 1**).

Trigeminal afferent loss yields neurotrophic keratopathy, a degenerative disease of the ocular surface.[4] The cornea and overlying tear film are key components of the ocular surface, and comprise the principal refractive optics of the visual system. Given its exposure, the ocular surface is prone to injury. Afferent neural input to the ocular surface provides critical regulatory and protective functions. The pathophysiology of neurotrophic keratopathy comprises a loss of sensory feedback and trophic support to the ocular surface. Sensory feedback regulates the protective blink and tearing reflexes in response to ocular foreign bodies and desiccation. Sensory branches of the trigeminal nerve also produce trophic neuropeptides that stimulate wound healing in response to injury and maintain the integrity of the ocular surface in the uninjured state.[5] Neuromediators released from corneal nerves are manifold, and include substance P, calcitonin gene-related peptide, neuropeptide Y, brain natriuretic peptide, vasointestinal

For submission to: Facial Plastic Surgery Clinics.
Financial Support: None.
[a] Department of Otolaryngology–Head & Neck Surgery, Massachusetts Eye and Ear, Harvard Medical School, 243 Charles Street, Boston, MA 02114, USA; [b] Department of Ophthalmology, Massachusetts Eye and Ear, Harvard Medical School, 243 Charles Street, Boston, MA 02114, USA
* Corresponding author.
E-mail address: nate_jowett@meei.harvard.edu

Facial Plast Surg Clin N Am 29 (2021) 459–470
https://doi.org/10.1016/j.fsc.2021.03.011

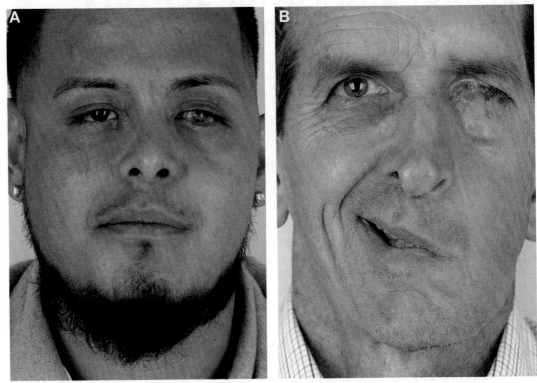

Fig. 1. Trigeminal anesthesia. (*A*) Left facial anesthesia secondary to a gunshot wound to the skull base 2 years prior. He developed advanced neurotrophic keratopathy with marked vision loss and resultant disfigurement on the affected side. (*B*) Combined facial paralysis and trigeminal anesthesia after extirpation of a large skull base vestibular schwannoma 2 years prior. The patient underwent permanent central tarsorrhaphy to protect his ocular surface, resulting in complete obstruction of the left visual field and further disfigurement.

peptide, and acetylcholine.[6] In turn, corneal epithelial cells and keratocytes regulate the survival and maturation of corneal nerve fibers by release of several neurotrophins and neuropeptides, including nerve growth factor, neutrohin-3 and neutrohin-4/5, brain-derived neurotrophic factor, and glial cell–derived neurotrophic factor.[7] Inadequate healing and progressive ocular surface degeneration in neurotrophic keratopathy may occur in the absence of mechanical insult, owing to morphologic and metabolic disturbances resulting from loss of trigeminal afferent neural trophic support.[8,9]

The clinical presentation of neurotrophic keratopathy ranges from subtle corneal surface irregularities to corneal melting or perforation (**Fig. 2**). Vision loss in neurotrophic keratopathy is insidious; erosion of the ocular surface occurs is painless owing to absence of sensory feedback. The disease is typically graded in 3 stages according to Mackie's classification.[10] Stage I is characterized by hyperplasia or irregularity of the corneal epithelium, evolving to punctate keratopathy, corneal edema, neovascularization, and stromal scarring. Stage II is defined by recurrent or persistent epithelial defects. In stage III,

stromal involvement leads to corneal ulceration, melting, and perforation. Concomitant facial paralysis and trigeminal anesthesia places patients at high risk of vision loss; paralytic lagophthalmos accelerates the progression of neurotrophic keratopathy.

Beyond corneal blindness, trigeminal anesthesia places the facial soft tissues at risk of injury. Biting of the lip, cheek, and tongue on the affected side occurs without nociceptive feedback. Absent vermillion sensation increases the propensity for oral incompetence and social embarrassment as food debris on the lips goes unnoticed.[11–13] A subset of patients with congenital or acquired trigeminal dysfunction will develop trigeminal trophic syndrome (**Fig. 3**).[14,15] This devastating condition is believed to be the result of self-traumatization of insensate regions of the involved hemiface, knowingly or unknowingly, in response to paresthesiae. The onset of trigeminal trophic syndrome may occur weeks to years after trigeminal nerve injury, although typically within 1 to 2 years.[16] The nasal base and nasal ala are commonly involved, and demonstrate crescenteric ulcerations.[16,17] Left untreated, the disease often results in complete destruction of the nasal ala and may also involve

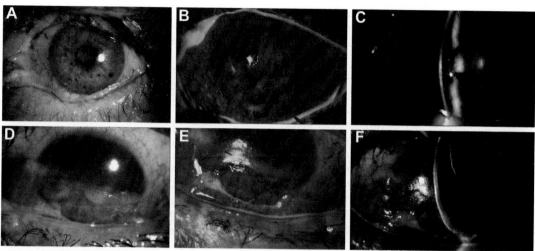

Fig. 2. Neurotrophic keratopathy. (*A–C*) Mackie stage I disease. Brightfield photography (*A*) demonstrates a fine haze over the ocular surface; diffuse conjunctival exudates and denudation of the upper eyelid gray line is also noted. Fluorescein fluorescence (*B*) and slit-lamp (*C*) examination demonstrate diffuse superficial punctate keratopathy without epithelial defect. (*D–F*) Mackie stage II disease. Brightfield photography (*D*) demonstrates global haze and inferior keratinization. Fluorescein fluorescence (*E*) and slit-lamp (*F*) examination demonstrates oval-shaped persistent epithelial defect.

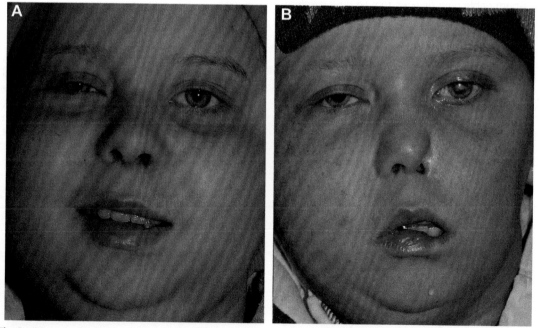

Fig. 3. Trigeminal trophic syndrome. The patient developed left trigeminal anesthesia and incomplete facial palsy after stereotactic radiotherapy to the skull base for the treatment of Ewing's sarcoma. (*A*) Two months after treatment, subtle erythema is noted about the left nasal vestibule. (*B*) Two years later, the patient returned with near-total loss of the left nasal ala, loss of left lower lip volume, and left neurotrophic keratitis with central clouding of the cornea.

the lips, cheek, forehead, and orbit on the affected side. Concurrent neurotrophic keratopathy is typical.

THERAPEUTIC MANAGEMENT OF NEUROTROPHIC KERATOPATHY
Medical Management

Therapeutic management of neurotrophic keratopathy aims to promote corneal healing while avoiding further insult to the ocular surface. Therapy of neurotrophic keratopathy depends on disease stage. In stage I disease, therapy aims to improve the integrity and transparency of the corneal epithelium and avoid further epithelial breakdown. Therapy involves the application of artificial tears during waking hours and gels or ointments overnight. Topical lubricants should be free of preservatives, because they may yield toxic or atopic keratoconjunctivitis.[18] Topical autologous serum and therapeutic soft contact lenses may be used for persistent keratopathy.

In stage II disease, therapy aims to promote the healing of persistent epithelial defects and prevent ulceration. In addition to stage I treatments, medical therapies may include topical recombinant human nerve growth factor administration (eg, cenegermin),[19] levator muscle chemodenervation, the judicious use of topical antibiotics and corticosteroids, and scleral lenses. Scleral lenses are gas-permeable rigid devices that lie on the sclera and vault over the cornea; prosthetic replacement of the ocular surface ecosystem devices are custom-tailored scleral lenses that may yield improved performance.[20] The disadvantages of rigid lenses include a heightened risk of microbial keratopathy and corneal hypoxia, yielding neovascularization.[21]

Therapy in stage III disease aims to promote ulcer healing and avoid perforation. In stage III, additional medical therapies may include topical N-acetylcysteine and systemic medroxyprogesterone or tetracycline in cases of corneal melt.[22,23] Surgical interventions are often indicated in stages II and III neurotrophic keratopathy owing to the limitations of medical therapy.

Surgical Management

Adjunctive surgical treatments
Surgical therapy of advanced neurotrophic keratopathy (stages II and III) is targeted at promoting healing of the ocular surface or replacing damaged or missing tissues. Decreasing ocular surface exposure through levator lengthening or tarsorrhaphy (lateral, medial, or central) establishes an optimal healing environment by minimizing desiccation and foreign body insult. The disadvantages of such procedures include poor aesthetics and decreased visual fields (**Fig. 4**). Where conservative measures have failed, adhesive therapy (cyanoacrylate or fibrin glue), conjunctival flap surgery, amniotic membrane transplantation, and lamellar or penetrating keratoplasty may be indicated. Corneal transplantation carries a high risk of failure in neurotrophic keratopathy where sensory neural input has not been reestablished (**Fig. 5**). When present, paralytic lagophthalmos should be addressed immediately using static periocular reanimation techniques and motor neurotization of the orbicularis oculi muscle where indicated.

Corneal neurotization
The management of neurotrophic keratopathy is challenging and costly.[24] Although conventional therapies may halt disease progression and stimulate corneal healing in neurotrophic keratopathy, they do not address its underlying cause. In 2009, Terzis and colleagues[25] demonstrated that

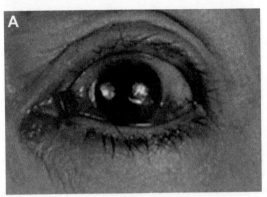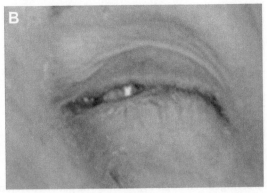

Fig. 4. Tarsorrhaphy for neurotrophic keratopathy. (*A*) The patient developed progressive neurotrophic keratopathy secondary to combined trigeminal anesthesia and paralytic lagophthalmos from a skull base Teflon granuloma occurring 15 years after microvascular decompression for trigeminal neuralgia. (*B*) Rapid progression of neurotrophic keratopathy was subsequently managed with central tarsorrhaphy to prevent corneal perforation.

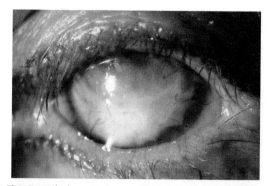

Fig. 5. Failed corneal transplant in neurotrophic keratopathy. The patient developed trigeminal anesthesia and advanced neurotrophic keratopathy after radiofrequency ablation of the trigeminal ganglion for the management of trigeminal neuralgia. Several months after penetrating keratoplasty, diffuse opacification of the allograft is noted. Corneal neurotization was subsequently performed and the patient is awaiting revision corneal transplant.

the progression of neurotrophic keratopathy could be reversed via by surgical transfer of contralateral supraorbital and supratrochlear nerve branches to the affected side perilimbal region. Widespread adaptation of this remarkable technique was initially hindered by its donor site morbidity and technical challenge, requiring a bicoronal incision and meticulous dissection of the terminal sensory nerve branches yielding anesthesia of the contralateral forehead. International interest in the approach was sparked when Elbaz and colleagues[26] and Bains and associates[27] described the use of an interposition nerve autograft between the cornea and donor supratrochlear nerve to decrease procedural morbidity.

Indications Indications for corneal neurotization have not been established definitively. In cases of acquired trigeminal anesthesia, there exists the potential for the spontaneous recovery of sensory function where the continuity of corneal nerve branches with the brainstem and cortex exists. Examples include recent-onset neurotrophic keratopathy secondary to herpes keratopathy and skull base surgery where anatomic continuity of the trigeminal nerve was preserved. In such cases, watchful waiting with conservative medical and surgical measures to protect the ocular surface should be considered for at least 1 year. Indications for corneal neurotization are clear in cases of advanced neurotrophic keratopathy (stages II and III) refractory to conservative measures where corneal anesthesia is complete and long standing. Because patients with corneal anesthesia are at

constant risk of rapid progression of neurotrophic keratopathy yielding corneal blindness, consideration of corneal neurotization is appropriate in all cases of corneal anesthesia without the potential for sensory recovery. In cases of long-standing corneal hypoesthesia (ie, some preserved sensation to the ocular surface), neurotization may be considered for neurotrophic keratopathy refractive to conservative measures. Corneal neurotization may yield particular benefit in patients with advanced cornea opacification, wherein the goal is to render them candidates for second-stage corneal transplant for vision restoration.

It is unknown whether corneal neurotization procedures impact the recovery of native corneal nerve function after a transient insult, although emerging data suggest alternate neurotization of the ocular surface may provide trophic support that enhances remnant corneal nerve function in cases of corneal hypoesthesia.[28] Anecdotal evidence suggests that nerve transfers may unmask remnant corneal nerve function in select cases. In our own experience, we have noted at least 1 patient with long-standing corneal anesthesia who recovered sensation localizing to the ocular surface in addition to the native dermatome of the donor nerve after corneal neurotization.

Approaches Corneal neurotization approaches vary according to donor nerve source, use and type of interposition graft, and the methods to secure the transferred nerve fascicles to the ocular surface. Donor nerve options in corneal neurotization procedures are dictated by the pattern of sensory loss noted on meticulous physical examination. Potential donor nerves include the contralateral supratrochlear, supraorbital branches, and ipsilateral great auricular nerve branches. In select cases, the ipsilateral supratrochlear, supraorbital, or infraorbital branches of the trigeminal nerve may be suitable for use. Corneal neurotization may be achieved via direct transposition of the distal segments of donor nerves or via the use of an interposition graft to bridge the gap between the donor neurotization source and the ocular surface. Owing to their length, ease of harvest, and low morbidity, sural nerve autografts are used commonly. The use of acellular nerve allografts in place of nerve autografts carries an increased risk of suboptimal neurotization in graft lengths exceeding 3 to 4 cm,[29–31] yet several centers have used them for corneal neurotization.[32] Transferred nerve fascicles are routed from the facial soft tissues to the subconjunctival space; they may be secured to the perilimbal sclera using microsutures or alternatively placed directly within the corneal stroma via scleral–corneal tunnels and secured using fibrin glue.[33]

Corneal neurotization procedures carry a favorable safety profile. In their pioneering work using a bicoronal approach, Terzis and colleagues[25] reported 1 subgaleal hematoma requiring drainage, and 1 asymptomatic subconjunctival neuroma requiring no treatment. Using an interposition graft to bridge the fibers of the contralateral supratrochlear nerve to the perilimbal region, Catapano and colleagues[34] reported conjunctival suture exposure in several patients where nylon sutures were used. Postoperative persistence of epithelial defects was also noted in several patients, all resolving with bandage contact lens therapy. No autograft donor site morbidity was encountered. In our center's experience (8 cases to date), we noted 1 case of persistent focal conjunctival chemosis that resolved with topical steroids and simple excision.

Outcome measures Clinical and research outcome measures in corneal neurotization are manifold. Clinical photography with slit-lamp examination with and without fluorescein together with assessment of visual acuity is regularly performed. Corneal sensation (native and referred) may be quantified and longitudinally tracked using Cochet–Bonnet esthesiometry.[35] In vivo corneal confocal microscopy may be used to visualize regenerating nerve fibers within the cornea (**Fig. 6**). Pachymetry may be used to assess corneal thickness. The histopathologic examination of explanted tissue obtained during subsequent corneal transplant procedures may confirm the presence of nerve fibers.[28] Noninvasive functional imaging of the brain during tactile stimulation of the ocular surface has been used in research settings to confirm transferred nerves yield sensation.[34]

The success of corneal neuortization is gauged principally on whether measurable sensory feedback has been reestablished, and whether visual acuity and integrity of the ocular surface remains stable or improves. Procedural success may depend on donor nerve axonal load, regeneration length and quality of the nerve graft where used, microsurgical technique, patient age and comorbidities, duration of corneal anesthesia, degree of remnant corneal nerve function, and stage of neurotrophic keratopathy. A recent review of published results identified 54 operated eyes, wherein significant improvement of best-corrected visual acuity (mean improvement of 0.41 logarithm of the minimum angle of resolution; standard deviation, 0.55; $P<.0001$) and central corneal sensation (mean improvement of 38.0 mm on esthesiometry; standard deviation, 18.95; $P<.0001$) after corneal neurotization.[36] The

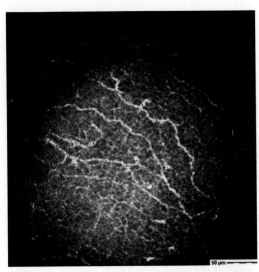

Fig. 6. In vivo corneal confocal microscopy. A 670-nm lower power laser scanning microscope generates confocal images of the anterior segment of the eye from backscattered and reflected light. Terminal branches of the corneal nerves are readily visualized within the highly transparent corneal stroma.

median time to the restoration of maximal sensation was 8 months.[36]

Technique Presently, our preferred approach for corneal neurotization is by transfer of the ipsilateral great auricular nerve to the ocular surface using a sural nerve autograft (**Fig. 7**). A 2-team approach is used; a cornea team prepares the ocular surface for receipt of the nerve fascicles while a microsurgical team harvests a long sural nerve graft. A small infra-auricular incision is made, and subplatysmal flaps elevated to expose anterior and posterior branches of the great auricular nerve on the affected side. Next, a sural nerve is harvested using an endoscope through a 1-inch incision posterior to the lateral malleolus. The larger caliber component of the sural nerve is used for interposition grafting, typically the medial cutaneous component.

Brimonidine is instilled onto the ocular surface. An eyelid speculum is placed, and a U-shaped inferior fornix-based peritomy constructed 7 mm posterior to the limbus (see **Fig. 7**A). Hemostasis is achieved using bipolar pencil cautery. A fascia needle is passed from the subconjunctival plane in the inferolateral fornix deep to the inferior tarsus into the subsuperficial musculoaponeurotic system plane of the cheek and out through the ipsilateral infra-auricular incision (see **Fig. 7**B).

The nerve autograft is secured using a vessel loop to the eye of the needle (see **Fig. 7**B), which is then withdrawn to interpose the graft between

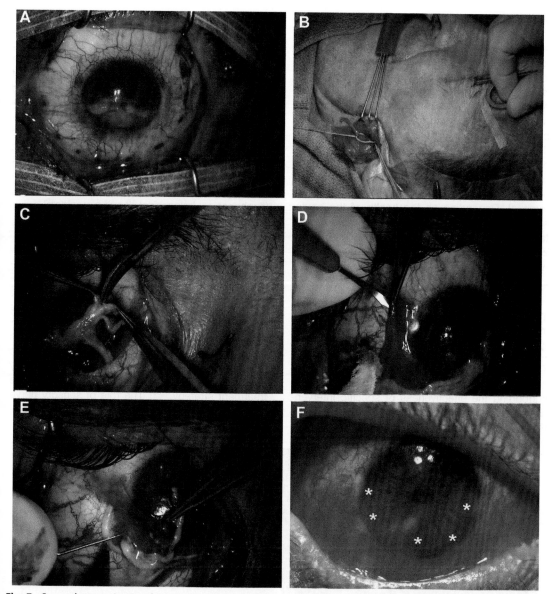

Fig. 7. Corneal neurotization by great auricular nerve transfer. (*A*) A U-shaped fornix-based conjunctival flap is designed and elevated to the limbus. (*B*) A fascia needle is passed from the subconjunctival space out an infra-auricular incision atop the terminal branches of the great auricular nerve. A sural nerve autograft is secured to the eyelet and interposed between the great auricular nerve and the ocular surface by withdrawal of the needle. (*C*) Interfascicular dissection of the graft is performed at the ocular surface to separate individual fascicles. (*D*) Scleral–corneal tunnels into the anterior corneal stroma are made for each fascicle about the limbus from 2 o'clock to 10 o'clock. (*E*) An Osher Y hook is used to position fascicle tips within the tunnels. The conjunctival flap is redraped, and fibrin glue instilled within the subconjunctival space to fix fascicles in position. (*F*) Five months after surgery, 5 fascicle tips (*) are visible within the anterior corneal stroma.

the donor nerve and the ocular surface. Under high stereoscopic magnification, interfascicular dissection is performed of the ocular end of the graft to separate individual nerve fascicles (typically 4–8) over a distance of 15 mm (see **Fig. 7**C). A crescent blade is used to create an equal number of scleral–corneal tunnels into the anterior corneal stroma,

spaced circumferentially around the inferior limbus between 2 o'clock and 10 o'clock (see **Fig. 7**D). The fascicle tips are trimmed to suitable length to allow full range of extraocular movements, and meticulously inserted into the scleral–corneal tunnels using an Osher Y hook (see **Fig. 7**E). The fornix-based conjunctival flap is redraped and fibrin glue applied subconjunctivally to seal the flap edges while securing fascicles into position. A temporary lateral suture tarsorrhaphy is then performed. Attention is turned to the infra-auricular incision. The other end of the interposition graft is trimmed to appropriate length and coapted to branches of the great auricular nerve using interrupted 10-0 nylon sutures, and the neck incision closed in 2 layers with absorbable sutures. Patients are discharged on the same day or after overnight observation with a 1-month tapering dose of ophthalmic tobramycin/dexamethasone, returning 2 weeks later for tarsorrhaphy suture removal. Depending on the health of the ocular surface, bandage contact lenses or permanent tarsorrhaphy may be used until adequate neurotization is noted. The fascicle tips may be seen within the corneal stroma about the limbus for several months after surgery (see **Fig. 7**F).

THERAPEUTIC MANAGEMENT OF TRIGEMINAL TROPHIC SYNDROME
Medical Management

The management of trigeminal trophic syndrome is challenging. Owing to its rarity, rigorous evidence supporting the effectiveness of specific interventions in trigeminal trophic syndrome is lacking. Recognition of the syndrome is a critical first step;

trigeminal nerve dysfunction is a hallmark of the disease. The differential diagnosis includes carcinoma, vasculitis, and pyoderma gangrenosum. Counseling is paramount; providing insight to patients as to the pathophysiology of the disease may suffice to halt self-induced trauma (**Fig. 8**). The use of hydrocolloid dressings and prostheses may protect ulcerated regions and dissuade ongoing unrecognized self-traumatization to allow healing.[16] Other proposed conservative treatments include transcutaneous electrical nerve stimulation,[37] antibiotics, gabapentin,[38] antidepressants (amitriptyline[39]), anticonvulsants (carbamazepine[40,41]), and neuroleptics (fluphenazine, haloperidol,[16] and pimozide[42]).

Surgical Management

Surgical interventions for trigeminal trophic syndrome are targeted at preventing ongoing self-induced trauma and reconstructing existing deficits. Cervical sympathectomy was reported effective in a single case report.[14] Long-term success with transposition of sensate regional flaps for reconstruction of nasal ala defects secondary to trigeminal trophic syndrome has been reported, suggesting sensory neurotization of affected regions may be an effective treatment strategy.[43,44] The role of sensory nerve transfer for management of trigeminal trophic syndrome has not been previously studied.

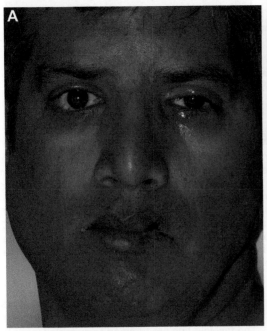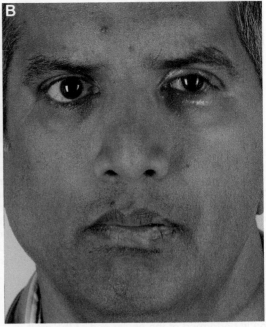

Fig. 8. Counseling in trigeminal trophic syndrome. (*A*) Ulceration of the left upper and lower lips is noted in this patient, 28 months after the onset of combined left facial paralysis and trigeminal anesthesia secondary to extirpation of a large vestibular schwannoma. The patient was diagnosed with trigeminal trophic syndrome and counseled to avoid digital trauma to the region. (*B*) One year later, resolution of lip ulcerations is noted with mild scarring and pigmentary changes.

THERAPEUTIC MANAGEMENT OF FACIAL ANESTHESIA
Medical Management

Few options exist in the medical management of facial anesthesia. In the acute setting, where the trigeminal nerve is believed to be anatomically intact, watchful waiting paired with counseling and conservative corneal protective measures with close ophthalmologic follow-up is indicated. Physical therapy with sensory reeducation may yield benefit.[45] Referral to a specialized pain clinic for management of dysesthesias when present is prudent.

Surgical Management

Where feasible, direct repair of the discontinuous trigeminal nerve branches should be considered. For example, lip anesthesia secondary to distal mental nerve injury may be addressed via direct nerve repair through an intraoral incision. Interposition nerve grafts should be used in all cases where direct end-to-end repair would necessitate tension. Where direct repair of the trigeminal nerve is not possible, for instance after a skull base surgery, sensory nerve transfer may be used for rehabilitation. Cross-mental nerve grafting may be used to restore mechanosensory function in an anesthetic lower hemilip.[46] Herein, sensory axons from a large terminal mental nerve branch on the healthy hemiface are transferred to a distal recipient stump on the affected side to neurotize the insensate lip, typically by means of an interposition nerve autograft. Recently, Catapano and colleagues[13] characterized

cross-infraorbital grafting paired with cross-mental grafting for sensory neurotization of upper and lower lips in trigeminal anesthesia, with an objective improvement in monofilament sensory testing noted at 4 months postoperatively. Herein, the authors used an epineurial window at the level of the infraorbital and mental nerve foramina for side-to-end coaptation of nerve grafts on the donor side, paired with end-to-end coaptation with respective nerve branches at the foramina on the affected side.

Technique

Our current approach prioritizes neurotization of the vermillion of the upper and lower lips, owing to their pivotal role in articulation and oral competence, as well as the risk of inadvertent injury with prandial activity. We use end-to-end interposition grafts between terminal branches to the vermillion on donor and recipient sides. Cross-mental and cross-infraorbital neurotization procedures may be performed concurrently with corneal neurotization, wherein harvest of a single sural nerve yields sufficient graft length for all 3 interpositions. Using this approach in 4 patients, we have documented the reestablishment of light touch sensation to the affected side within 4 months of nerve grafting, with touch perceived on the healthy side. Donor nerve harvest has not yielded noticeable loss of sensation on the healthy side lips on light touch and pinprick examination.

For the lower lip,[47] 2 small transverse incisions are made in the inferior vestibule and terminal mental nerve branches coursing through the plane between the minor salivary glands and orbicularis oris muscle are identified. One or 2 sizable terminal

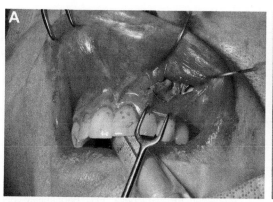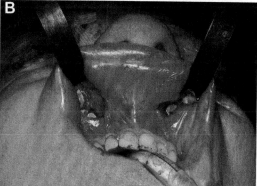

Fig. 9. Cross-infraorbital nerve grafting for sensory neurotization of the upper lip. Two small transverse incisions are made in the vestibule of the upper lip and terminal mental nerve branches identified. (A) Two large terminal infraorbital nerve branches to the vermillion of the healthy side upper lip are used as donor source for sensory axons. (B) A small interposition nerve graft is tunneled across the upper lip to a coalescence of terminal branches to the affected side vermillion. End-to-end coaptation of the graft is performed between vermillion branches under high stereoscopic magnification, and incisions closed in a single layer using chromic suture. The procedure was combined with corneal neurotization and cross-mental nerve grafting for sensory neurotization of the lower lip using a single long sural nerve autograft.

branches to the vermillion on the healthy side are used as donors. Donor branches are transected sharply distally and coapted to a short interposition graft tunneled within the submucosal plane to the affected side. Terminal mental nerve branches to the vermillion on the affected side are identified and traced proximally to identify their coalescence, which is then transected sharply and reflected superiorly for coaptation to the interposition graft.

The approach is similar for the upper lip (**Fig. 9**). Two small transverse incisions are made in the superior vestibule and terminal infraorbital nerve branches coursing atop the orbicularis oris muscle are identified. One or 2 sizable terminal branches to the vermillion on the healthy side are sharply transected and routed to a coalescence of terminal branches to the affected side vermillion via a short interposition nerve graft tunneled across the upper lip.

DISCUSSION

Mounting evidence suggests a role for nerve transfers in the rehabilitation of trigeminal anesthesia. The surgical transfer of a regional sensory nerve to circumvent the loss of native afferent input to a critical target is analogous to the transfer of regional motor axons to restore critical motor function, such as hypoglossal transfer in cases of facial paralysis. Owing to the preponderance of muscle toward decreased receptivity to neurotization over time, motor nerve transfers are generally contraindicated for denervation periods exceeding 1 to 2 years. There exists no equivalent time limit when contemplating sensory nerve transfers, especially where fresh nerve autografts are used for direct sensory neurotization of a distal target. In cases of neurotrophic keratopathy, benefit from sensory nerve transfer has been reported among patients with corneal anesthesia in excess of 20 years before corneal neurotization.[25]

Multicenter randomized controlled trials are required to compare the effectiveness of corneal neurotization in comparison to medical therapy including topical recombinant human nerve growth factor in early stage neurotrophic keratopathy. Facial sensory neurotization techniques require further study using objective quantified metrics and validated patient-reported outcome measures to characterize their effectiveness. The role of cross-facial sensory neurotization in the management of recalcitrant trigeminal trophic syndrome warrants study. Basic research into the mechanisms of cranial nerve regeneration to identify novel therapeutic targets to optimize rehabilitative outcomes in nerve transfers is critical to advance the field. Specialized fellowships to train the next generation of surgeons in these emerging techniques would yield societal benefit.

SUMMARY

Trigeminal anesthesia yields devastating functional and aesthetic sequelae. An increasing number of therapeutic options are emerging to relieve suffering for patients stricken with this rare disease.

CLINICS CARE POINTS

- Trigeminal anesthesia may yield neurotrophic keratopathy, functional impairment in the oral phase of deglutition, and trigeminal trophic syndrome.
- Concomitant paralytic lagophthalmos and trigeminal anesthesia may cause rapid corneal blindness.
- Emerging evidence supports a role for corneal neurotization in the management of neurotrophic keratopathy.
- Candidacy criteria and optimal surgical strategies for corneal neurotization require further clarification.
- Acellular nerve allografts have demonstrated inferiority to nerve autografts over distances in excess of 3 to 4 cm in animal and human studies.
- Progression of trigeminal trophic syndrome may be halted with prompt diagnosis and counseling.
- Surgical strategies for sensory neurotization of the facial soft tissues require further study using rigorous outcome measures.

DISCLOSURE

The authors have nothing to disclose.

REFERENCES

1. Schneider ER, Gracheva EO, Bagriantsev SN. Evolutionary Specialization of Tactile Perception in Vertebrates. Physiology (Bethesda) 2016;31(3): 193–200.
2. Humphrey T. Some correlations between the appearance of human fetal reflexes and the development of the nervous system. Progress in brain research. New York: Elsevier; 1964. p. 93–135.

3. Ardiel EL, Rankin CH. The importance of touch in development. Paediatr Child Health 2010;15(3):153–6.

4. Bonini S, Rama P, Olzi D, et al. Neurotrophic keratopathy. Eye 2003;17(8):989–95.

5. Reid TW, Murphy CJ, Iwahashi CK, et al. Stimulation of epithelial cell growth by the neuropeptide substance P. J Cell Biochem 1993;52(4):476–85.

6. Mastropasqua L, Massaro-Giordano G, Nubile M, et al. Understanding the pathogenesis of neurotrophic keratopathy: the role of corneal nerves. J Cell Physiol 2017;232(4):717–24.

7. You L, Kruse FE, Völcker HE. Neurotrophic Factors in the Human Cornea. Invest Ophthalmol Vis Sci 2000;41(3):692–702.

8. Muller LJ, Marfurt CF, Kruse F, et al. Corneal nerves: structure, contents and function. Exp Eye Res 2003;76(5):521–42.

9. Magendie F. De l'influence de la cinquieme paire de nerfs sur la nutrition et les fonctions de l'oeil. J Physiol Exp Pathol 1824;4:176–82.

10. Mackie I, Fraunfelder F. Current ocular therapy. 4th edition. Philadelphia, PA: WB Saunders; 1995. p. 506–8.

11. Calverley JR, Mohnac AM. Syndrome of the Numb Chin. Arch Intern Med 1963;112:819–21.

12. Lee EG, Ryan FS, Shute J, et al. The impact of altered sensation affecting the lower lip after orthognathic treatment. J Oral Maxillofac Surg 2011;69(11):e431–45.

13. Catapano J, Scholl D, Ho E, et al. Restoration of trigeminal cutaneous sensation with cross-face sural nerve grafts: a novel approach to facial sensory rehabilitation. Plast Reconstr Surg 2015;136(3):568–71.

14. McKenzie K. Observations on the results of the operative treatment of trigeminal neuralgia. Can Med Assoc J 1933;29(5):492.

15. Loveman AB. An unusual dermatosis following section of the fifth cranial nerve. Arch Dermatol Syphilol 1933;28(3):369–75.

16. Dicken CH. Trigeminal trophic syndrome. Mayo Clin Proc 1997;72(6):543–5.

17. Sadeghi P, Papay FA, Vidimos AT. Trigeminal trophic syndrome—report of four cases and review of the literature. Dermatol Surg 2004;30(5):807–12.

18. Baudouin C. Detrimental effect of preservatives in eyedrops: implications for the treatment of glaucoma. Acta Ophthalmol 2008;86(7):716–26.

19. Lambiase A, Rama P, Bonini S, et al. Topical treatment with nerve growth factor for corneal neurotrophic ulcers. N Engl J Med 1998;338(17):1174–80.

20. Chahal JS, Heur M, Chiu GB. Prosthetic replacement of the ocular surface ecosystem scleral lens therapy for exposure keratopathy. Eye Contact Lens 2017;43(4):240–4.

21. Walker MK, Bergmanson JP, Miller WL, et al. Complications and fitting challenges associated with scleral contact lenses: a review. Cont Lens Anterior Eye 2016;39(2):88–96.

22. Hicks CR, Crawford GJ. Melting after keratoprosthesis implantation: the effects of medroxyprogesterone. Cornea 2003;22(6):497–500.

23. Hossain P. The corneal melting point. Eye 2012;26(8):1029–30.

24. Sacchetti M, Lambiase A. Diagnosis and management of neurotrophic keratopathy. Clin Ophthalmol (Auckland, NZ) 2014;8:571–9.

25. Terzis JK, Dryer MM, Bodner BI. Corneal neurotization: a novel solution to neurotrophic keratopathy. Plast Reconstr Surg 2009;123(1):112–20.

26. Elbaz U, Bains R, Zuker RM, et al. Restoration of corneal sensation with regional nerve transfers and nerve grafts: a new approach to a difficult problem. JAMA Ophthalmol 2014;132(11):1289–95.

27. Bains RD, Elbaz U, Zuker RM, et al. Corneal neurotization from the supratrochlear nerve with sural nerve grafts: a minimally invasive approach. Plast Reconstr Surg 2015;135(2):397e–400e.

28. Ting DSJ, Figueiredo GS, Henein C, et al. Corneal neurotization for neurotrophic keratopathy: clinical outcomes and in vivo confocal microscopic and histopathological findings. Cornea 2018;37(5):641–6.

29. Jowett N, Pineda Ii R. Acellular nerve allografts in corneal neurotisation: an inappropriate choice. Br J Ophthalmol 2020;104(2):149–50.

30. Hong T, Wood I, Hunter DA, et al. Neuroma management: capping nerve injuries with an acellular nerve allograft can limit axon regeneration. Hand 2019. https://doi.org/10.1177/1558944719849115. 1558944719849115.

31. Leckenby JI, Furrer C, Haug L, et al. A retrospective case series reporting the outcomes of advanced nerve allografts in the treatment of peripheral nerve injuries. Plast Reconstr Surg 2020;145(2):368e–81e.

32. Sweeney AH, Wang M, Weller CL, et al. Outcomes of corneal neurotisation using processed nerve allografts: a multicentre case series. Br J Ophthalmol 2020. https://doi.org/10.1136/bjophthalmol-2020-317361. bjophthalmol-2020-317361.

33. Jowett N, Pineda RI. Corneal neurotization by great auricular nerve transfer and scleral-corneal tunnel incisions for neurotrophic keratopathy. Br J Ophthalmol 2018;103(9):1235–8.

34. Catapano J, Fung SSM, Halliday W, et al. Treatment of neurotrophic keratopathy with minimally invasive corneal neurotisation: long-term clinical outcomes and evidence of corneal reinnervation. Br J Ophthalmol 2019. https://doi.org/10.1136/bjophthalmol-2018-313042. bjophthalmol-2018-313042.

35. Cochet P, Bonnet R. Anesthésie corneenne. Clin Ophthalmol 1960;4:3–27.

36. Park JK, Charlson ES, Leyngold I, et al. Corneal neurotization: a review of pathophysiology and

outcomes. Ophthal Plast Reconstr Surg 2020;36(5):431–7.

37. Westerhof W, Bos J. Trigeminal trophic syndrome: a successful treatment with transcutaneous electrical stimulation. Br J Dermatol 1983;108(5):601–4.

38. Garza I. The trigeminal trophic syndrome: an unusual cause of face pain, dysaesthesias, anaesthesia and skin/soft tissue lesions. Cephalalgia 2008;28(9):980–5.

39. Finlay AY. Trigeminal trophic syndrome. Arch Dermatol 1979;115(9):1118.

40. Fruhauf J, Schaider H, Massone C, et al. Carbamazepine as the only effective treatment in a 52-year-old man with trigeminal trophic syndrome. Mayo Clin Proc 2008;83(4):502–4.

41. Bhushan M, Parry EJ, Telfer NR. Trigeminal trophic syndrome: successful treatment with carbamazepine. Br J Dermatol 1999;141(4):758–9.

42. Mayer R, Smith N. Improvement of trigeminal neurotrophic ulceration with pimozide in a cognitively impaired elderly woman—a case report. Clin Exp Dermatol 1993;18(2):171–3.

43. Abyholm FE, Eskeland G. Defect of the ala nasi following trigeminal denervation. Case report. Scand J Plast Reconstr Surg 1977;11(1):87–90.

44. McLean NR, Watson AC. Reconstruction of a defect of the ala nasi following trigeminal anaesthesia with an innervated forehead flap. Br J Plast Surg 1982;35(2):201–3.

45. Meyer RA, Bagheri SC. Nerve injuries from mandibular third molar removal. Atlas Oral Maxillofac Surg Clin North Am 2011;19(1):63–78.

46. Kaban LB, Upton J. Cross mental nerve graft for restoration of lip sensation after inferior alveolar nerve damage: report of case. J Oral Maxillofac Surg 1986;44(8):649–51.

47. Mohan S, Jowett N. Motor and sensory rehabilitation of the lower lip. Oper Tech Otolaryngol Head Neck Surg 2020;31(1):45–54.

Moving?

Make sure your subscription moves with you!

To notify us of your new address, find your **Clinics Account Number** (located on your mailing label above your name), and contact customer service at:

Email: journalscustomerservice-usa@elsevier.com

800-654-2452 (subscribers in the U.S. & Canada)
314-447-8871 (subscribers outside of the U.S. & Canada)

Fax number: 314-447-8029

Elsevier Health Sciences Division
Subscription Customer Service
3251 Riverport Lane
Maryland Heights, MO 63043

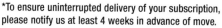
*To ensure uninterrupted delivery of your subscription, please notify us at least 4 weeks in advance of move.

ELSEVIER

Printed and bound by CPI Group (UK) Ltd, Croydon, CR0 4YY

08/05/2025

01864692-0007